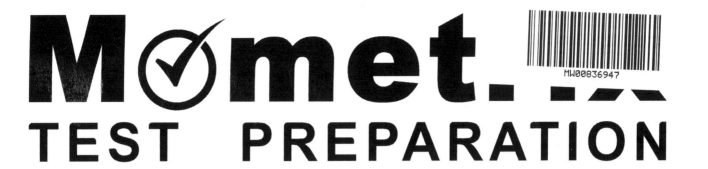

Mometrix
TEST PREPARATION

MW00836947

Secrets of the
Orthodontic Assisting
Exam Study Guide

DEAR FUTURE EXAM SUCCESS STORY

First of all, **THANK YOU** for purchasing Mometrix study materials!

Second, congratulations! You are one of the few determined test-takers who are committed to doing whatever it takes to excel on your exam. **You have come to the right place.** We developed these study materials with one goal in mind: to deliver you the information you need in a format that's concise and easy to use.

In addition to optimizing your guide for the content of the test, we've outlined our recommended steps for breaking down the preparation process into small, attainable goals so you can make sure you stay on track.

We've also analyzed the entire test-taking process, identifying the most common pitfalls and showing how you can overcome them and be ready for any curveball the test throws you.

Standardized testing is one of the biggest obstacles on your road to success, which only increases the importance of doing well in the high-pressure, high-stakes environment of test day. Your results on this test could have a significant impact on your future, and this guide provides the information and practical advice to help you achieve your full potential on test day.

Your success is our success

We would love to hear from you! If you would like to share the story of your exam success or if you have any questions or comments in regard to our products, please contact us at **800-673-8175** or **support@mometrix.com**.

Thanks again for your business and we wish you continued success!

Sincerely,
The Mometrix Test Preparation Team

Need more help? Check out our flashcards at:
http://MometrixFlashcards.com/DANB

TABLE OF CONTENTS

Introduction

Thank you for purchasing this resource! You have made the choice to prepare yourself for a test that could have a huge impact on your future, and this guide is designed to help you be fully ready for test day. Obviously, it's important to have a solid understanding of the test material, but you also need to be prepared for the unique environment and stressors of the test, so that you can perform to the best of your abilities.

For this purpose, the first section that appears in this guide is the **Secret Keys**. We've devoted countless hours to meticulously researching what works and what doesn't, and we've boiled down our findings to the five most impactful steps you can take to improve your performance on the test. We start at the beginning with study planning and move through the preparation process, all the way to the testing strategies that will help you get the most out of what you know when you're finally sitting in front of the test.

We recommend that you start preparing for your test as far in advance as possible. However, if you've bought this guide as a last-minute study resource and only have a few days before your test, we recommend that you skip over the first two Secret Keys since they address a long-term study plan.

If you struggle with **test anxiety**, we strongly encourage you to check out our recommendations for how you can overcome it. Test anxiety is a formidable foe, but it can be beaten, and we want to make sure you have the tools you need to defeat it.

1

Secret Key #1 – Plan Big, Study Small

There's a lot riding on your performance. If you want to ace this test, you're going to need to keep your skills sharp and the material fresh in your mind. You need a plan that lets you review everything you need to know while still fitting in your schedule. We'll break this strategy down into three categories.

Information Organization

Start with the information you already have: the official test outline. From this, you can make a complete list of all the concepts you need to cover before the test. Organize these concepts into groups that can be studied together, and create a list of any related vocabulary you need to learn so you can brush up on any difficult terms. You'll want to keep this vocabulary list handy once you actually start studying since you may need to add to it along the way.

Time Management

Once you have your set of study concepts, decide how to spread them out over the time you have left before the test. Break your study plan into small, clear goals so you have a manageable task for each day and know exactly what you're doing. Then just focus on one small step at a time. When you manage your time this way, you don't need to spend hours at a time studying. Studying a small block of content for a short period each day helps you retain information better and avoid stressing over how much you have left to do. You can relax knowing that you have a plan to cover everything in time. In order for this strategy to be effective though, you have to start studying early and stick to your schedule. Avoid the exhaustion and futility that comes from last-minute cramming!

Study Environment

The environment you study in has a big impact on your learning. Studying in a coffee shop, while probably more enjoyable, is not likely to be as fruitful as studying in a quiet room. It's important to keep distractions to a minimum. You're only planning to study for a short block of time, so make the most of it. Don't pause to check your phone or get up to find a snack. It's also important to **avoid multitasking**. Research has consistently shown that multitasking will make your studying dramatically less effective. Your study area should also be comfortable and well-lit so you don't have the distraction of straining your eyes or sitting on an uncomfortable chair.

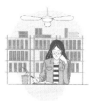 The time of day you study is also important. You want to be rested and alert. Don't wait until just before bedtime. Study when you'll be most likely to comprehend and remember. Even better, if you know what time of day your test will be, set that time aside for study. That way your brain will be used to working on that subject at that specific time and you'll have a better chance of recalling information.

Finally, it can be helpful to team up with others who are studying for the same test. Your actual studying should be done in as isolated an environment as possible, but the work of organizing the information and setting up the study plan can be divided up. In between study sessions, you can discuss with your teammates the concepts that you're all studying and quiz each other on the details. Just be sure that your teammates are as serious about the test as you are. If you find that your study time is being replaced with social time, you might need to find a new team.

2

Secret Key #2 – Make Your Studying Count

You're devoting a lot of time and effort to preparing for this test, so you want to be absolutely certain it will pay off. This means doing more than just reading the content and hoping you can remember it on test day. It's important to make every minute of study count. There are two main areas you can focus on to make your studying count.

Retention

It doesn't matter how much time you study if you can't remember the material. You need to make sure you are retaining the concepts. To check your retention of the information you're learning, try recalling it at later times with minimal prompting. Try carrying around flashcards and glance at one or two from time to time or ask a friend who's also studying for the test to quiz you.

To enhance your retention, look for ways to put the information into practice so that you can apply it rather than simply recalling it. If you're using the information in practical ways, it will be much easier to remember. Similarly, it helps to solidify a concept in your mind if you're not only reading it to yourself but also explaining it to someone else. Ask a friend to let you teach them about a concept you're a little shaky on (or speak aloud to an imaginary audience if necessary). As you try to summarize, define, give examples, and answer your friend's questions, you'll understand the concepts better and they will stay with you longer. Finally, step back for a big picture view and ask yourself how each piece of information fits with the whole subject. When you link the different concepts together and see them working together as a whole, it's easier to remember the individual components.

Finally, practice showing your work on any multi-step problems, even if you're just studying. Writing out each step you take to solve a problem will help solidify the process in your mind, and you'll be more likely to remember it during the test.

Modality

Modality simply refers to the means or method by which you study. Choosing a study modality that fits your own individual learning style is crucial. No two people learn best in exactly the same way, so it's important to know your strengths and use them to your advantage.

For example, if you learn best by visualization, focus on visualizing a concept in your mind and draw an image or a diagram. Try color-coding your notes, illustrating them, or creating symbols that will trigger your mind to recall a learned concept. If you learn best by hearing or discussing information, find a study partner who learns the same way or read aloud to yourself. Think about how to put the information in your own words. Imagine that you are giving a lecture on the topic and record yourself so you can listen to it later.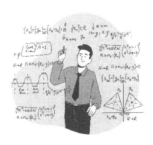

For any learning style, flashcards can be helpful. Organize the information so you can take advantage of spare moments to review. Underline key words or phrases. Use different colors for different categories. Mnemonic devices (such as creating a short list in which every item starts with the same letter) can also help with retention. Find what works best for you and use it to store the information in your mind most effectively and easily.

Secret Key #3 – Practice the Right Way

Your success on test day depends not only on how many hours you put into preparing, but also on whether you prepared the right way. It's good to check along the way to see if your studying is paying off. One of the most effective ways to do this is by taking practice tests to evaluate your progress. Practice tests are useful because they show exactly where you need to improve. Every time you take a practice test, pay special attention to these three groups of questions:

- The questions you got wrong
- The questions you had to guess on, even if you guessed right
- The questions you found difficult or slow to work through

This will show you exactly what your weak areas are, and where you need to devote more study time. Ask yourself why each of these questions gave you trouble. Was it because you didn't understand the material? Was it because you didn't remember the vocabulary? Do you need more repetitions on this type of question to build speed and confidence? Dig into those questions and figure out how you can strengthen your weak areas as you go back to review the material.

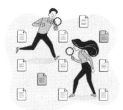 Additionally, many practice tests have a section explaining the answer choices. It can be tempting to read the explanation and think that you now have a good understanding of the concept. However, an explanation likely only covers part of the question's broader context. Even if the explanation makes perfect sense, **go back and investigate** every concept related to the question until you're positive you have a thorough understanding.

As you go along, keep in mind that the practice test is just that: practice. Memorizing these questions and answers will not be very helpful on the actual test because it is unlikely to have any of the same exact questions. If you only know the right answers to the sample questions, you won't be prepared for the real thing. **Study the concepts** until you understand them fully, and then you'll be able to answer any question that shows up on the test.

It's important to wait on the practice tests until you're ready. If you take a test on your first day of study, you may be overwhelmed by the amount of material covered and how much you need to learn. Work up to it gradually.

On test day, you'll need to be prepared for answering questions, managing your time, and using the test-taking strategies you've learned. It's a lot to balance, like a mental marathon that will have a big impact on your future. Like training for a marathon, you'll need to start slowly and work your way up. When test day arrives, you'll be ready.

Start with the strategies you've read in the first two Secret Keys—plan your course and study in the way that works best for you. If you have time, consider using multiple study resources to get different approaches to the same concepts. It can be helpful to see difficult concepts from more than one angle. Then find a good source for practice tests. Many times, the test website will suggest potential study resources or provide sample tests.

Practice Test Strategy

If you're able to find at least three practice tests, we recommend this strategy:

UNTIMED AND OPEN-BOOK PRACTICE

Take the first test with no time constraints and with your notes and study guide handy. Take your time and focus on applying the strategies you've learned.

TIMED AND OPEN-BOOK PRACTICE

Take the second practice test open-book as well, but set a timer and practice pacing yourself to finish in time.

TIMED AND CLOSED-BOOK PRACTICE

Take any other practice tests as if it were test day. Set a timer and put away your study materials. Sit at a table or desk in a quiet room, imagine yourself at the testing center, and answer questions as quickly and accurately as possible.

Keep repeating timed and closed-book tests on a regular basis until you run out of practice tests or it's time for the actual test. Your mind will be ready for the schedule and stress of test day, and you'll be able to focus on recalling the material you've learned.

Secret Key #4 – Pace Yourself

Once you're fully prepared for the material on the test, your biggest challenge on test day will be managing your time. Just knowing that the clock is ticking can make you panic even if you have plenty of time left. Work on pacing yourself so you can build confidence against the time constraints of the exam. Pacing is a difficult skill to master, especially in a high-pressure environment, so **practice is vital**.

Set time expectations for your pace based on how much time is available. For example, if a section has 60 questions and the time limit is 30 minutes, you know you have to average 30 seconds or less per question in order to answer them all. Although 30 seconds is the hard limit, set 25 seconds per question as your goal, so you reserve extra time to spend on harder questions. When you budget extra time for the harder questions, you no longer have any reason to stress when those questions take longer to answer.

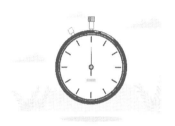

Don't let this time expectation distract you from working through the test at a calm, steady pace, but keep it in mind so you don't spend too much time on any one question. Recognize that taking extra time on one question you don't understand may keep you from answering two that you do understand later in the test. If your time limit for a question is up and you're still not sure of the answer, mark it and move on, and come back to it later if the time and the test format allow. If the testing format doesn't allow you to return to earlier questions, just make an educated guess; then put it out of your mind and move on.

On the easier questions, be careful not to rush. It may seem wise to hurry through them so you have more time for the challenging ones, but it's not worth missing one if you know the concept and just didn't take the time to read the question fully. Work efficiently but make sure you understand the question and have looked at all of the answer choices, since more than one may seem right at first.

Even if you're paying attention to the time, you may find yourself a little behind at some point. You should speed up to get back on track, but do so wisely. Don't panic; just take a few seconds less on each question until you're caught up. Don't guess without thinking, but do look through the answer choices and eliminate any you know are wrong. If you can get down to two choices, it is often worthwhile to guess from those. Once you've chosen an answer, move on and don't dwell on any that you skipped or had to hurry through. If a question was taking too long, chances are it was one of the harder ones, so you weren't as likely to get it right anyway.

On the other hand, if you find yourself getting ahead of schedule, it may be beneficial to slow down a little. The more quickly you work, the more likely you are to make a careless mistake that will affect your score. You've budgeted time for each question, so don't be afraid to spend that time. Practice an efficient but careful pace to get the most out of the time you have.

6

Secret Key #5 – Have a Plan for Guessing

When you're taking the test, you may find yourself stuck on a question. Some of the answer choices seem better than others, but you don't see the one answer choice that is obviously correct. What do you do?

The scenario described above is very common, yet most test takers have not effectively prepared for it. Developing and practicing a plan for guessing may be one of the single most effective uses of your time as you get ready for the exam.

In developing your plan for guessing, there are three questions to address:

- When should you start the guessing process?
- How should you narrow down the choices?
- Which answer should you choose?

When to Start the Guessing Process

Unless your plan for guessing is to select C every time (which, despite its merits, is not what we recommend), you need to leave yourself enough time to apply your answer elimination strategies. Since you have a limited amount of time for each question, that means that if you're going to give yourself the best shot at guessing correctly, you have to decide quickly whether or not you will guess.

Of course, the best-case scenario is that you don't have to guess at all, so first, see if you can answer the question based on your knowledge of the subject and basic reasoning skills. Focus on the key words in the question and try to jog your memory of related topics. Give yourself a chance to bring the knowledge to mind, but once you realize that you don't have (or you can't access) the knowledge you need to answer the question, it's time to start the guessing process.

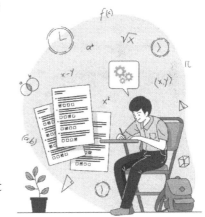

It's almost always better to start the guessing process too early than too late. It only takes a few seconds to remember something and answer the question from knowledge. Carefully eliminating wrong answer choices takes longer. Plus, going through the process of eliminating answer choices can actually help jog your memory.

Summary: Start the guessing process as soon as you decide that you can't answer the question based on your knowledge.

7

How to Narrow Down the Choices

The next chapter in this book (**Test-Taking Strategies**) includes a wide range of strategies for how to approach questions and how to look for answer choices to eliminate. You will definitely want to read those carefully, practice them, and figure out which ones work best for you. Here though, we're going to address a mindset rather than a particular strategy.

Your odds of guessing an answer correctly depend on how many options you are choosing from.

Number of options left	5	4	3	2	1
Odds of guessing correctly	20%	25%	33%	50%	100%

You can see from this chart just how valuable it is to be able to eliminate incorrect answers and make an educated guess, but there are two things that many test takers do that cause them to miss out on the benefits of guessing:

- Accidentally eliminating the correct answer
- Selecting an answer based on an impression

We'll look at the first one here, and the second one in the next section.

To avoid accidentally eliminating the correct answer, we recommend a thought exercise called **the $5 challenge**. In this challenge, you only eliminate an answer choice from contention if you are willing to bet $5 on it being wrong. Why $5? Five dollars is a small but not insignificant amount of money. It's an amount you could afford to lose but wouldn't want to throw away. And while losing

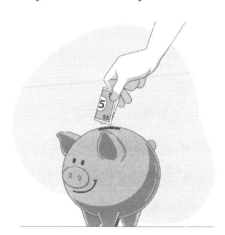

$5 once might not hurt too much, doing it twenty times will set you back $100. In the same way, each small decision you make—eliminating a choice here, guessing on a question there—won't by itself impact your score very much, but when you put them all together, they can make a big difference. By holding each answer choice elimination decision to a higher standard, you can reduce the risk of accidentally eliminating the correct answer.

The $5 challenge can also be applied in a positive sense: If you are willing to bet $5 that an answer choice *is* correct, go ahead and mark it as correct.

Summary: Only eliminate an answer choice if you are willing to bet $5 that it is wrong.

8

Which Answer to Choose

You're taking the test. You've run into a hard question and decided you'll have to guess. You've eliminated all the answer choices you're willing to bet $5 on. Now you have to pick an answer. Why do we even need to talk about this? Why can't you just pick whichever one you feel like when the time comes?

The answer to these questions is that if you don't come into the test with a plan, you'll rely on your impression to select an answer choice, and if you do that, you risk falling into a trap. The test writers know that everyone who takes their test will be guessing on some of the questions, so they intentionally write wrong answer choices to seem plausible. You still have to pick an answer though, and if the wrong answer choices are designed to look right, how can you ever be sure that you're not falling for their trap? The best solution we've found to this dilemma is to take the decision out of your hands entirely. Here is the process we recommend:

Once you've eliminated any choices that you are confident (willing to bet $5) are wrong, select the first remaining choice as your answer.

Whether you choose to select the first remaining choice, the second, or the last, the important thing is that you use some preselected standard. Using this approach guarantees that you will not be enticed into selecting an answer choice that looks right, because you are not basing your decision on how the answer choices look.

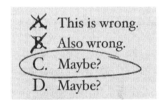

This is not meant to make you question your knowledge. Instead, it is to help you recognize the difference between your knowledge and your impressions. There's a huge difference between thinking an answer is right because of what you know, and thinking an answer is right because it looks or sounds like it should be right.

Summary: To ensure that your selection is appropriately random, make a predetermined selection from among all answer choices you have not eliminated.

Test-Taking Strategies

This section contains a list of test-taking strategies that you may find helpful as you work through the test. By taking what you know and applying logical thought, you can maximize your chances of answering any question correctly!

It is very important to realize that every question is different and every person is different: no single strategy will work on every question, and no single strategy will work for every person. That's why we've included all of them here, so you can try them out and determine which ones work best for different types of questions and which ones work best for you.

Question Strategies

ⵀ READ CAREFULLY

Read the question and the answer choices carefully. Don't miss the question because you misread the terms. You have plenty of time to read each question thoroughly and make sure you understand what is being asked. Yet a happy medium must be attained, so don't waste too much time. You must read carefully and efficiently.

ⵀ CONTEXTUAL CLUES

Look for contextual clues. If the question includes a word you are not familiar with, look at the immediate context for some indication of what the word might mean. Contextual clues can often give you all the information you need to decipher the meaning of an unfamiliar word. Even if you can't determine the meaning, you may be able to narrow down the possibilities enough to make a solid guess at the answer to the question.

ⵀ PREFIXES

If you're having trouble with a word in the question or answer choices, try dissecting it. Take advantage of every clue that the word might include. Prefixes can be a huge help. Usually, they allow you to determine a basic meaning. *Pre-* means before, *post-* means after, *pro-* is positive, *de-* is negative. From prefixes, you can get an idea of the general meaning of the word and try to put it into context.

ⵀ HEDGE WORDS

Watch out for critical hedge words, such as *likely, may, can, sometimes, often, almost, mostly, usually, generally, rarely,* and *sometimes*. Question writers insert these hedge phrases to cover every possibility. Often an answer choice will be wrong simply because it leaves no room for exception. Be on guard for answer choices that have definitive words such as *exactly* and *always*.

ⵀ SWITCHBACK WORDS

Stay alert for *switchbacks*. These are the words and phrases frequently used to alert you to shifts in thought. The most common switchback words are *but, although,* and *however*. Others include *nevertheless, on the other hand, even though, while, in spite of, despite,* and *regardless of*. Switchback words are important to catch because they can change the direction of the question or an answer choice.

10

⊘ Face Value

When in doubt, use common sense. Accept the situation in the problem at face value. Don't read too much into it. These problems will not require you to make wild assumptions. If you have to go beyond creativity and warp time or space in order to have an answer choice fit the question, then you should move on and consider the other answer choices. These are normal problems rooted in reality. The applicable relationship or explanation may not be readily apparent, but it is there for you to figure out. Use your common sense to interpret anything that isn't clear.

Answer Choice Strategies

⊘ Answer Selection

The most thorough way to pick an answer choice is to identify and eliminate wrong answers until only one is left, then confirm it is the correct answer. Sometimes an answer choice may immediately seem right, but be careful. The test writers will usually put more than one reasonable answer choice on each question, so take a second to read all of them and make sure that the other choices are not equally obvious. As long as you have time left, it is better to read every answer choice than to pick the first one that looks right without checking the others.

⊘ Answer Choice Families

An answer choice family consists of two (in rare cases, three) answer choices that are very similar in construction and cannot all be true at the same time. If you see two answer choices that are direct opposites or parallels, one of them is usually the correct answer. For instance, if one answer choice says that quantity x increases and another either says that quantity x decreases (opposite) or says that quantity y increases (parallel), then those answer choices would fall into the same family. An answer choice that doesn't match the construction of the answer choice family is more likely to be incorrect. Most questions will not have answer choice families, but when they do appear, you should be prepared to recognize them.

⊘ Eliminate Answers

Eliminate answer choices as soon as you realize they are wrong, but make sure you consider all possibilities. If you are eliminating answer choices and realize that the last one you are left with is also wrong, don't panic. Start over and consider each choice again. There may be something you missed the first time that you will realize on the second pass.

⊘ Avoid Fact Traps

Don't be distracted by an answer choice that is factually true but doesn't answer the question. You are looking for the choice that answers the question. Stay focused on what the question is asking for so you don't accidentally pick an answer that is true but incorrect. Always go back to the question and make sure the answer choice you've selected actually answers the question and is not merely a true statement.

⊘ Extreme Statements

In general, you should avoid answers that put forth extreme actions as standard practice or proclaim controversial ideas as established fact. An answer choice that states the "process should be used in certain situations, if..." is much more likely to be correct than one that states the "process should be discontinued completely." The first is a calm rational statement and doesn't even make a definitive, uncompromising stance, using a hedge word *if* to provide wiggle room, whereas the second choice is far more extreme.

⊘ Benchmark

As you read through the answer choices and you come across one that seems to answer the question well, mentally select that answer choice. This is not your final answer, but it's the one that will help you evaluate the other answer choices. The one that you selected is your benchmark or standard for judging each of the other answer choices. Every other answer choice must be compared to your benchmark. That choice is correct until proven otherwise by another answer choice beating it. If you find a better answer, then that one becomes your new benchmark. Once you've decided that no other choice answers the question as well as your benchmark, you have your final answer.

⊘ Predict the Answer

Before you even start looking at the answer choices, it is often best to try to predict the answer. When you come up with the answer on your own, it is easier to avoid distractions and traps because you will know exactly what to look for. The right answer choice is unlikely to be word-for-word what you came up with, but it should be a close match. Even if you are confident that you have the right answer, you should still take the time to read each option before moving on.

General Strategies

⊘ Tough Questions

If you are stumped on a problem or it appears too hard or too difficult, don't waste time. Move on! Remember though, if you can quickly check for obviously incorrect answer choices, your chances of guessing correctly are greatly improved. Before you completely give up, at least try to knock out a couple of possible answers. Eliminate what you can and then guess at the remaining answer choices before moving on.

⊘ Check Your Work

Since you will probably not know every term listed and the answer to every question, it is important that you get credit for the ones that you do know. Don't miss any questions through careless mistakes. If at all possible, try to take a second to look back over your answer selection and make sure you've selected the correct answer choice and haven't made a costly careless mistake (such as marking an answer choice that you didn't mean to mark). This quick double check should more than pay for itself in caught mistakes for the time it costs.

⊘ Pace Yourself

It's easy to be overwhelmed when you're looking at a page full of questions; your mind is confused and full of random thoughts, and the clock is ticking down faster than you would like. Calm down and maintain the pace that you have set for yourself. Especially as you get down to the last few minutes of the test, don't let the small numbers on the clock make you panic. As long as you are on track by monitoring your pace, you are guaranteed to have time for each question.

⊘ Don't Rush

It is very easy to make errors when you are in a hurry. Maintaining a fast pace in answering questions is pointless if it makes you miss questions that you would have gotten right otherwise. Test writers like to include distracting information and wrong answers that seem right. Taking a little extra time to avoid careless mistakes can make all the difference in your test score. Find a pace that allows you to be confident in the answers that you select.

⏱ Keep Moving

Panicking will not help you pass the test, so do your best to stay calm and keep moving. Taking deep breaths and going through the answer elimination steps you practiced can help to break through a stress barrier and keep your pace.

Final Notes

The combination of a solid foundation of content knowledge and the confidence that comes from practicing your plan for applying that knowledge is the key to maximizing your performance on test day. As your foundation of content knowledge is built up and strengthened, you'll find that the strategies included in this chapter become more and more effective in helping you quickly sift through the distractions and traps of the test to isolate the correct answer.

Now that you're preparing to move forward into the test content chapters of this book, be sure to keep your goal in mind. As you read, think about how you will be able to apply this information on the test. If you've already seen sample questions for the test and you have an idea of the question format and style, try to come up with questions of your own that you can answer based on what you're reading. This will give you valuable practice applying your knowledge in the same ways you can expect to on test day.

Good luck and good studying!

14

Evaluation

Examination

PATIENT RECORDS COMPONENTS

Patient records are legal documents that include all pertinent information related to the individual and his or her care.

- These records should contain a patient registration form that documents all important demographic information, such as patient name, address, phone numbers, employer, spousal information, data about the responsible party (if different) who is accountable for payment, insurance information if applicable (including a copy of the insurance card), and chief reason for the visit
- Another very important section of a patient's record is a comprehensive medical history, including points that address issues that can affect care, such as medication history (prescription as well as over-the-counter), radiation exposure, and identified allergies
- If the patient has a condition that could affect care, a brightly colored medical alert sticker should be visible inside the patient record
- The record should also contain a dental history form, which should be authorized by the dentist
- All forms should be signed and dated by the patient

PATIENT FORMS

If the patient has any conditions that may require consultation with his or her physician, the individual must sign a release of information form.

- All patients should be informed in writing of the right to privacy under the Health Insurance Portability and Accountability Act (HIPAA); after signing, these forms should be kept for at least 6 years
- Before subsequent visits, patients should be required to bring their medical history up to date on an update form
- Other data that should be included in the patient's record are laboratory reports pertinent to the person's medical history, including tests for infectious diseases such as hepatitis or human immunodeficiency virus (HIV)
- Any information gleaned through examination, dental charting, or oral radiography should also be documented

PATIENT VITAL SIGNS

Vital signs are part of the patient's preliminary physical examination.

- Vital signs should also be taken at subsequent visits and should be documented immediately
- They include body temperature, pulse rate, respiration rate, and blood pressure
- Body temperature is usually taken orally with a digital thermometer
- Pulse rate, which expresses heart beat at various arteries, should be taken by placing the index and middle (or possibly additional) fingers on one of the patient's pulse locations and then counting

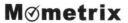

- These points could be either the radial (inner wrist on thumb side), carotid (groove of neck on side of trachea), brachial (antecubital space below bend of elbow on inner arm), or temporal (depression between eyebrow and ear)
- Respiration rate, which indicates efficiency of oxygen intake and carbon dioxide output, is approximated by observation by watching the rise and fall of the patient's chest
- One respiration is a breath taken in followed by one let out (inhalation followed by exhalation)
- Often respirations are observed while the technician keeps his or her fingers on the radial pulse site to relax the patient

BLOOD PRESSURE

Blood pressure is related to the work required by the heart to pump blood. There are two components of blood pressure (BP) measurement, systolic and diastolic.

- These components are usually expressed as a ratio of systolic to diastolic (that is, systolic/diastolic)
- Systolic pressure is a measurement of the contraction of the heart, during which it pumps oxygenated blood to the arteries from the left chamber of the heart
- The diastolic pressure is a reflection of the heart during expansion when it fills up with blood returning from the body to be oxygenated
- BP can be taken using either an automated electronic blood pressure device or a stethoscope and sphygmomanometer in combination

BLOOD PRESSURE PROCEDURE

The patient is seated with an arm held out at heart level.

- Usually the brachial artery (lower inner arm) pulse rate should be manually determined first and added to 40 to determine the inflation level for the sphygmomanometer
- For example, a pulse rate of 80 beats a minute suggests inflation up to 120 mm mercury (Hg)
- The sphygmomanometer consists of a cuff that is attached to a rubber bulb regulated by a valve that controls blood flow and a manometer for pressure readings
- The cuff is wrapped around the arm
- Air in the cuff is forced out by opening the valve
- The cuff is wrapped so that it fits fairly closely around the patient's arm about 1 inch above the antecubital space (the inside of the arm above the elbow)
- The healthcare professional then places the stethoscope earpieces in his or her ears and its disc over the brachial artery
- Using the other hand, he or she rapidly inflates the cuff using the rubber bulb to the aforementioned setting
- He or she listens through the stethoscope while gradually releasing the valve
- When an initial distinct thumping is heard, the systolic pressure is recorded; when sounds cease, the diastolic pressure is noted
- Two readings are taken
- Earpieces should be disinfected after use

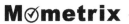

NORMAL VITAL SIGNS

Body temperature should be between 96.0 and 99.5 (average 98.6) degrees Fahrenheit or 35.5 to 37.5 (average 37.0) degrees Celsius.

- Readings above these indicate the presence of a fever, which can often be alleviated through use of cold packs, alcohol rubs, or aspirin
- Lower temperatures indicate hypothermia from cold exposure or use of aspirin or other antipyretics

Adults normally have a pulse rate of 60 to 90 beats a minute and children 90 to 120 beats a minute (70-110 in other texts).

- Higher and lower resting pulse rates are called tachycardia and bradycardia
- There are also other possible abnormalities, such as an irregular heart beat (arrhythmia)

Respiration rates should be between 10 to 20 breaths a minute for adults and 18 to 30 breaths for children (other sources indicate 12-18 for adults and 20-40 for children).

- Unusually high or low resting rates are known as tachypnea and bradypnea respectively

Normal BP levels are 100 to 140 mm Hg for the systolic component and 60 to 90 mm Hg for the diastolic component; the average adult BP is 120/80 and adolescent BP is often higher.

- High blood pressure or hypertension indicates abnormally hard work on the part of the heart, especially if the diastolic reading is high
- Low blood pressure is termed hypotension

EXTERNAL CLINICAL EVALUATION

The dental assistant should scrutinize the patient as he or she enters the room for any indications of abuse, nutrition issues, or abnormalities associated with health problems or aging.

- Abnormalities that can specifically impact dental or orthodontic care and should be noted are exaggerated facial asymmetry, swelling, speech problems or habits, and behaviors, such as mouth breathing or thumb sucking.
- The clinical evaluation should include an examination of patient's lips for cracking or parching.
- The assistant should also examine the smile line where lips meet, the peripheral vermillion border line of the lip, and the lip corners or commissures.
- With the lips closed, the assistant then checks the mandible and external floor of the mouth by external palpation.
- As the patient turns his or her head to the side, the cervical lymph nodes between the ear and collar bone are similarly examined usually from behind.
- The patient's temporomandibular joint (TMJ) is inspected externally; the assistant sits behind the individual and palpates in front the tragus of the ear while the patient opens and closes the mouth to identify any clicking noises, snagging, or pain.

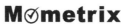

INTERNAL CLINICAL EVALUATION

After the prospective dental patient is examined extraorally, an internal oral examination is done.

- Mouth wounds, abscessed teeth, and abnormal colorations of the mucosa are noted
- The dentist or assistant should then hold the mandible in one hand and palpate the underside of the tongue and the floor of the mouth with the fingers
- The oral mucosa and frenum (fold) are examined by pulling the lips outward, generally from behind
- A mouth mirror is used to inspect the buccal or cheek area
- The tongue is also examined with the mirror
- This includes pulling it to the side and upward with gauze to facilitate full observation
- The patient is instructed to say "ah" as a means of inspecting the entrance to the throat and the tissues of the oropharynx
- A certified dental or orthodontic assistant can legally perform the external and internal clinical evaluation in most states
- In addition, the dentist uses a hand instrument to prod the hard surface of every tooth, and the assistant notes any findings in the patient's record

CHARTING COMPONENTS

Tooth diagrams are usually either anatomic or geometric.

- An anatomic diagram has pictures that look like real teeth possibly including the roots
- A geometric diagram uses circles to represent each tooth, and the circle is divided to signify different tooth surfaces
- Each chart has positions for all 16 upper and 16 lower teeth
- There are several different numbering systems that might be used, most notably the Universal/National System
- The teeth are shown as if one is looking into the individual's mouth
- Information about completed dental treatments is indicated in either blue or black on the chart, and newly detected or uncompleted treatments are noted in red
- Cavities are noted on the diagram and chart as Classes I to VI using Black's classification as the standard
- Dental offices may use a variety of symbols or short forms to describe conditions or materials used in the patient's mouth on his or her chart

UNIVERSAL/NATIONAL SYSTEM

In the United States, the Universal/National System sanctioned by the American Dental Association is generally used to number teeth.

- Permanent teeth are designated by numbers 1 through 32 starting with the upper-right third molar as tooth #1 and proceeding along the top to tooth #16 or the upper-left third molar
- The lower teeth are numbered starting at the lower left third molar as tooth #17 and ending at tooth #32 or the lower-right third molar

- Primary teeth are identified by letters A through J in the upper jaw from the right second molar to the left second molar, and the mandibular teeth are lettered from K through T starting with the left second molar and ending with the right second molar

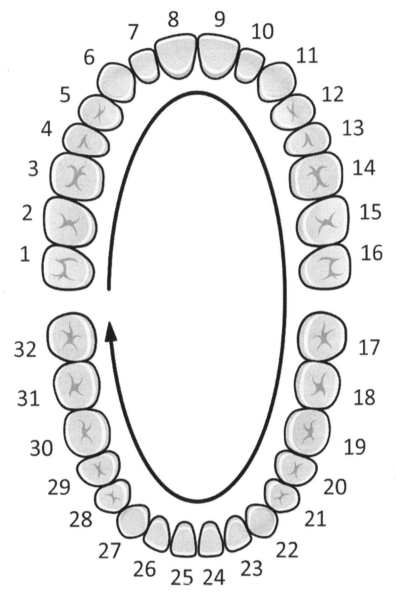

ALTERNATIVE TOOTH NUMBERING SYSTEMS

Outside the United States, most countries utilize the International Standards Organization System/Federation Dentaire Internationale (ISO/FDI).

- This system uses 2 digits, the first describing the quadrant and the second the tooth in that quadrant starting in the center
- The first digit for permanent teeth is 1, 2, 3, or 4 for the right maxillary, left maxillary, left mandibular, and right mandibular quadrants respectively
- The second digit in each quadrant runs from 1 through 8 starting at the center
- Primary teeth also are numbered by a 2-digit system, utilizing the quadrant followed by the tooth number starting at the center

- Here the quadrants are numbered from 5 through 8 as above, and the second digit only goes from 1 through 5 as there are fewer teeth
- In each, the digits are articulated separately
- Alternatively, the Palmer Notation System uses brackets (vertical line on one side plus a horizontal line below or above) around a number for permanent teeth or a letter for primary teeth to delineate the quadrant
- The number representing the tooth proceeds from the center from 1 through 8 for permanent teeth and the letters for primary ones go from A through E

DENTAL ARCHES AND QUADRANTS

Dentition is the normal arrangement of teeth in the mouth.

- Teeth are positioned into one of two dental arches
- Teeth set into the maxilla bone comprise the upper maxillary arch; this arch is affixed to the skull
- The lower teeth are situated in the mandible bone and comprise the mandibular arch, which has more flexibility to move around
- If positioned correctly, adjoining teeth touch each other and those in the maxillary arch contact and slightly overlap those in the mandibular arch when brought together
- Dental quadrants are areas of dentition defined by the arch they are in and whether they are to the right or left side of the midline dividing sides of the face
- There are 4 dental quadrants: maxillary right quadrant, maxillary left quadrant, mandibular right quadrant, and mandibular left quadrant
- The primary or deciduous teeth normally grown initially by children should number 20 so that there are 5 in each quadrant
- The permanent teeth developed later are normally 32 in number with 8 in each quadrant

DECIDUOUS AND PERMANENT DENTITION

The deciduous (or primary) teeth that develop initially in children should number 20 (10 in each arch, 5 in each quadrant). Each quadrant normally contains the following teeth starting at the midline and extending toward the back:

- (1) central incisor
- (2) lateral incisor (both utilized for cutting)
- (3) canine or cuspid (used to tear food)
- (4) first molar
- (5) second molar (both molars employed for chewing)
- When complete, the permanent teeth number 32 (16 per arch, 8 per quadrant)

From the midline to the back of each arch, the permanent teeth in each quadrant are as follows:

- (1) central incisor
- (2) lateral incisor
- (3) canine (all with functions similar to primary teeth)
- (4) first premolar
- (5) second premolar (premolars, also called bicuspids, used to chop up food)
- (6) first molar
- (7) second molar
- (8) third molar (all used to chew food)

- In both types of dentition, the central incisor, lateral incisor, and canine teeth are referred to as anterior teeth and have single roots and a distinct incisal edge
- For both types of dentition, the teeth further back are referred to as posterior teeth and have more than one root and cusp (grinding surface)

ERUPTION AND EXFOLIATION SCHEDULE

Primary or deciduous dentition starts erupting at about 6 months of age and is generally complete by the time the child is about 32 months old.

- The eruption schedule is fairly similar for both the maxillary and mandibular arch with the order of eruption being the central incisors, followed by the lateral incisors, the first molars, the canines, and the second molars
- The primary teeth are cast off from the oral cavity or exfoliated in approximately the same order
- Exfoliation generally starts at age 6 to 7, beginning with the central incisor
- The process should be complete by 10 to 12 years of age with the canines and second molars shed last

PERMANENT DENTITION ERUPTION SCHEDULE

From about the age of 6 to 12, a child has mixed dentition because permanent begin to erupt during this period before all primary teeth have been shed.

- The permanent teeth that eventually replace the central incisors, lateral incisors, and canines are said to be succedaneous (they succeed deciduous teeth)
- The molars are not succedaneous, and in fact, the first molars are generally the first permanent teeth
- They appear in both arches at about 6 to 7 years of age
- These teeth are followed by the central incisors and lateral incisors in both arches
- The other teeth may come in differently for the two arches
- The second and third molars are the last teeth to come in (usually in by age 13 and 21 respectively)

TEETH DIVISIONS AND SURFACES

Each tooth has a crown enclosed by enamel, a root faced with a thin layer of bony tissue called cementum, and a cervical line (the cementoenamel junction) dividing the two.

- The anatomical and clinical crowns and roots can differ as anatomical describes the actual covering material and clinical refers to the portion of that component that is discernible in the mouth
- The front or anterior teeth have 5 surfaces on the crown:
  - (1) mesial, facing the midline
  - (2) distal, facing away from the midline
  - (3) labial, exterior opposite the lips
  - (4) lingual, interior in the direction of the tongue (also known as palatal for the maxillary teeth)
  - (5) incisal or cutting-edge
- The back or posterior teeth also have 5 surfaces on the crown:
  - (1) mesial
  - (2) distal

- o (3) lingual (all as described above)
- o (4) buccal, exterior toward the cheek
- o (5) occlusal, the top chewing surface
- Another term for labial or buccal surfaces is facial
- Surfaces are either convex (curving outward), concave (curving inward), or flat, and any combination can be found on the same tooth

TEETH ANATOMICAL STRUCTURES

Anatomical landmarks used to identify teeth include the following:

- (1)Bifurcation or trifurcation: These are defined as 2 or 3 roots coming from main trunk of the tooth; the dividing spot is known as a furcation
- (2) Grooves or depressions: These are 3 types of grooves (depressions), buccal grooves, developmental grooves on the occlusal surface, or supplemental grooves emanating from the developmental type; fissures are imperfectly united developmental grooves, and pits are areas where fissures come together
- (3) Ridges: Ridges are elevated sections of enamel; the 4 types are marginal, oblique, transverse, and triangular; only marginal ridges are found on anterior teeth, whereas all types can be observed on molars
- (4) Fossa: Fossa are relatively superficial rounded or angular depressions
- (5) Apex: The apex is at or near the terminus of the root; the apical foramen is an opening at the apex through which nerves and blood vessels come into the tooth
- (6) Cusp: A cusp is a mound on the crown of the tooth; most molars have multiple cusps; the first molars may also have a fifth cusp on the mesial lingual surface known as the Cusp of Carabelli; lobes are partitions that unite to form teeth (usually equivalent to cusps for molars)
- (7) Cingulum: The cingulum is a convex space on lingual surface of the front teeth
- (8) Mamelons: These are three protuberances on the incisal edge of new central incisors

ANTERIOR MAXILLARY TEETH

The maxillary incisors have sharp incisal edges but no cusps.

- They have single roots, which are up to two times the length of the crown
- The maxillary central incisors near the midline are slightly larger (both crown and root) than the adjacent maxillary lateral incisors
- When central incisors initially erupt, they display three bumps on the incisal surface called mamelons, which eventually wear down to form a flat edge
- They usually also have imbrication or faint overlapping lines and developmental depressions on the labial surface near the gums
- The labial surface of the crown curves outward while the lingual side is primarily concave
- Incisors are essential for producing certain speech sounds
- Maxillary lateral incisors often vary from the expected
- The maxillary canines (cuspids) have the longest roots in the maxillary arch, making them the most secure
- The labial surface of the crown is convex with a vertical ridge while the incisal edge comes to a tip; the lingual side has two hollow fossas separated by a ridge and other ridges
- Canines contain more dentin (calcium-containing material) below the enamel, making them look darker

POSTERIOR MAXILLARY TEETH

The maxillary first and second premolars or bicuspids (posterior to canines) both have crowns with two cusps.

- For each, the facial cusp on the crown is larger than the lingual one, but the difference is more pronounced in the first premolar
- Maxillary first premolars have two bifurcated roots, whereas the maxillary second premolars have single roots
- Proceeding posteriorly, the maxillary first molars come next
- These teeth are almost square in shape and have 5 cusps
- The cusps are mesio-buccal, disto-buccal, mesio-lingual, disto-lingual, and the cusp of Carabelli, which is on the mesio-lingual cusp
- There is a buccal groove between the mesio-buccal and disto-buccal cusps as well as buccal and lingual pits, a central fossa, and oblique and transverse ridges
- Maxillary first molars have trifurcated roots
- Maxillary second molars are slightly smaller and have only four cusps (missing the cusp of Carabelli); they have trifurcated roots
- Maxillary third molars are a bit slighter than the second molars and have more grooves on the occlusal surface
- Their root structure can vary
- These molars may be absent or fail to erupt, indicating removal

ANTERIOR MANDIBULAR TEETH

Contrary to dentition in the maxillary arch, the mandibular central incisor is smaller than the adjoining lateral incisor.

- Mandibular central incisors have single, very straight, pointed roots
- The crowns are very slender and sharp at the edge (initial mamelons wear off), and they have convex labial and concave lingual surfaces and a cingulum
- The only differences in the lateral incisors are larger crowns with relatively smaller distal sides and smaller single roots that may have concave surfaces
- The mandibular canines or bicuspids have single roots with deep depressions; they may be shorter than those of the equivalent teeth in the upper arch
- The crowns have steeping sloping distal cusps and smaller mesial cusps

POSTERIOR MANDIBULAR TEETH

The mandibular first premolar (or bicuspid) has two cusps on the crown, the more prominent buccal cusp, and the relatively diminutive lingual cusp with an occlusal groove between.

- There are mesial, distal, and transverse ridges
- These premolars have short, straight single roots
- The mandibular second premolar has up to three short lingual cusps and one buccal cusp
- There are three grooves and ridges on the occlusal surface
- They have one root that angles a bit distally
- The mandibular first molars are the biggest teeth in the mouth
- They have five cusps meeting on the occlusal face in a central fossa with grooves in between each set of cusps
- The crown is somewhat concave on the mesial side but is quite straight distally
- This pattern is somewhat reflected in the two root structure (mesial and distal) as well

- The mesial root has two separate pulp canals
- The mandibular second molar is smaller than the first with four cusps meeting on the occlusal surface with grooves plus buccal and lingual grooves that terminate in pits or depressions
- Second molars usually have bifurcated roots
- Mandibular third molars, if they erupt, are smaller with multiple roots and a furrowed surface

DECIDUOUS MAXILLARY TEETH

In general, deciduous or primary teeth have relatively long roots compared to their crowns, more prominent cervical ridges, and a more whitish coloration (due thin enamel and dentin and more pulp).

- All deciduous teeth are usually smaller than later permanent teeth
- The maxillary deciduous central incisors have distinct cervical lines; they are wider than their height, and there are no mamelons as with initial permanent teeth; the labial side is flat and convex
- The maxillary deciduous lateral incisors are smaller, longer, and more curved than the central incisors
- The maxillary deciduous canines or cuspids have pointed incisal rims, ridges on the mesial and distal sides, and a prominent cingulum
- Their roots are more elongated than the incisors
- All of these anterior teeth have single roots
- The maxillary deciduous first molars have four cusps (with the mesio-lingual one being the most prominent), transverse and oblique ridges, and three roots
- The second molars have four main cusps (and possibly a fifth) and three widely separated roots

DECIDUOUS MANDIBULAR TEETH

The mandibular deciduous central incisor is very similar to its permanent equivalent except that the crown is a bit wider and both lingual and labial surfaces are curved while the sides are flat.

- The mandibular deciduous lateral incisors are slightly longer and broader than the central incisors; they have a prominent cingulum, distal and mesial ridges, and a deeper fossa
- Their roots bend distally at the bottom
- The mandibular deciduous canines are distinguished by smaller roots and less prominent crown ridges than their maxillary counterparts
- Mandibular deciduous incisors and canines have single roots
- The mandibular deciduous first molars have four cusps (with mesio-buccal being the biggest), relatively long buccal facades, and bifurcated roots on the mesial and distal sides
- The mandibular deciduous second molars look much like the permanent mandibular first molars but smaller
- However, the mesio-buccal and disto-buccal cusps are about the same size, it has two roots with the mesial one being bigger than the distal one

INFLAMMATION

Inflammation is the body's reaction to infection or injury.

- The process is clinically characterized by redness, heat, swelling, and pain
- Inflammation occurs because an injury or disease causes specialized immune cells to release chemicals, notably histamine, into the area
- The histamine causes increased blood flow, manifesting as redness and heat, and elevated amounts of blood
- The blood can seep from the capillaries into surrounding tissues, causing distension
- If nearby nerve endings are affected, a pain response also takes place. In addition, white blood cells are recruited to the vicinity to kill microorganisms, and a fibrous connective tissue network may surround the area
- The dental or orthodontic assistant should be attuned to the signs of inflammation as they represent some underlying disease process
- In the mouth, inflammation can be observed as a variety of lesions on the surface of the oral mucosa

ABOVE SURFACE OF THE ORAL MUCOSA

Oral lesions that might be observed above the surface of the oral mucosa include blisters, bullas, pustules, vesicles, papules, plaques, and hematomas.

- Blisters are fluid-containing elevated areas
- The fluid is the result of leakage from blood vessels as a result of trauma
- Vesicles, bullas, and pustules are all variations of blisters characterized respectively by small size, large size (a diameter larger than 0.5 inch), or pus within the blister
- Hematomas are reddish lesions containing a semi-solid mass of blood from a ruptured blood vessel; they are commonly observed after application of oral anesthetic
- A plaque is any elevated (or level) lesion in the oral mucosa

UNDERNEATH SURFACE OF THE ORAL MUCOSA

Oral lesions that might be observed underneath the surface of the oral mucosa include abscesses, cysts, ulcers, and erosions.

- Abscesses are pus-filled cavities resulting from bacterial infection and inflammation; in the oral cavity, they are generally found near the apex of the tooth or in the periodontal area
- Cysts are cavities that contain fluid or a semi-solid, fluid mixture; cyst formation can be related to many causes, most notably in the mouth from duct blockage
- Ulcers occur when mucous membranes are damaged and appear as reddened, painful, open sores
- Erosions are the indentations left after trauma; they have red and tender borders

FLAT SURFACE OF THE ORAL MUCOSA

There are a number of types of oral lesions that might be observed flat on the surface of the oral mucosa, including macules, ecchymosis, patches, petechiae, purpura, granulomas, neoplasms, and nodules.

- The latter three may also present above the surface of the oral mucosa
- Macules and patches are spots and areas respectively that differ in texture and/or color from their surroundings

25

- Ecchymosis refers to bruising of tissues
- Hemorrhaging can produce petechiae, small red or purple spots, or purpura, which is a more inclusive term that includes petechiae and larger areas of discoloration up to an inch in diameter that could be considered tissue bruising
- Neoplasms are tumorous growths, either benign or malignant
- A granuloma is one type of neoplasm in which there is chronic inflammation producing an area of granulation tissue
- Nodules are small protuberances of either hard or soft tissue

ORAL DISEASES AND LESIONS BACTERIA

The most common bacterial infections associated with oral diseases are actinomycosis and syphilis.

- Actinomycosis is caused by Actinomyces israelii; it initially manifests as painful swelling, which is followed by pus and yellow granules
- The primarily venereal disease syphilis, caused by infection with Treponema pallidum, has 3 stages that have oral consequences as well
- Lip chancres, firm and raised lesions that develop ulcers and crusting, occur in the first stage of syphilis
- Second and third stage syphilis are characterized by infectious patches or papules and localized gummas or tumors respectively
- Children of mothers with the disease can have tooth enamel hypoplasia or some other variation of this, such as Hutchinson's incisor's (ragged incisal edges) or mulberry molars

VIRUSES OR FUNGI ORAL LESIONS

The most common oral lesions associated with viral infections are from the herpes viruses.

- Oral lesions may result from infection with herpes simplex types I or II or herpes zoster
- Herpes simplex type I is primarily found in mouth lesions, but type II (the primarily genital variation) may also be found in these lesions
- Herpes simplex is spread through physical contact, usually initially during childhood, but eruptions can occur throughout life
- Herpes simplex oral lesions have a vesicular and crusted stage and appear as painful, inflamed blisters or cold sores on the lips or in the oral cavity
- Dental personnel should avoid or take infectious precautions when dealing with patients with outbreaks as they can develop ulcers on their fingers or hands if infected
- Herpes zoster or shingles is a reactivation of childhood varicella or chickenpox; the lesions are usually one-sided, painful, and long-lasting
- Individuals with HIV are predisposed toward herpes zoster or abnormally long bouts of herpes simplex
- Candidiasis, or thrush, is a yeast infection characterized orally by a thick, white layer over the mucous membranes; it can be treated by wiping the area and applying topical antifungal drugs

APHTHOUS ULCERS

Aphthous ulcers, also known as canker sores, are painful oral ulcerations of unknown origin characterized by lesions that have yellow centers encircled by red halos.

- The yellow center is actually necrosis of epithelial cells
- These ulcers do not appear to be contagious

- Causative agents have not been identified, but streptococci have often been found, and other factors such as stress, hormonal changes, food allergies, or stress appear to play a role
- Aphthous ulcers generally recur periodically and typically persist for about 10 to 14 days
- They can be soothed with topical anesthetics
- Oral procedures may need to be postponed during exacerbations as they are very painful

ORAL TRAUMA AND LESIONS

Oral trauma and lesions are generally caused by a dental procedure, radiation injury, or self-induced trauma.

- Dental instruments if used incorrectly can tear or bruise the oral mucosa
- Incorrect removal of cotton rolls used to dry tissue can induce ulcers in the gums
- Ulcers can also be initiated through irritation from improperly fitting dentures, in these cases, folds of extra tissue called hyperplasia eventually form and the palate develops red, swollen lumps
- When amalgam is used for dental procedures, particles can get caught in tissue, turning the area blue or gray, fortunately, this so-called amalgam tattoo poses no health issue
- Excess radiation delivered to the oral cavity is usually associated with head and neck cancer therapies and can cause teeth to lose their roots or become misshapen
- Radiation can also cause ulcers in the area
- Self-induced traumas to the oral cavity usually result from such things as biting the inside of the cheek or prodding the tissue with a dull object

TOBACCO

Tobacco use is one of the main chemical causes of oral lesions.

- Nicotine stomatitis is common in pipe smokers and, to lesser extent, in cigarette smokers
- Areas that are repeatedly exposed to the heat and chemicals in tobacco smoke initially show redness from irritation and then develop white and red hyperkeratinized or excessively thick bumps containing keratin
- The person's salivary gland openings may also become inflamed. Another type of tobacco-related lesion can occur with use of snuff or chewing tobacco
- The lesion occurs generally in the lower front area between the lips and the teeth and is similar to other nicotine stomatitis
- Irritations from smoking marijuana can look very similar, although they usually occur inside both lips

CHEMICAL AGENTS

So-called hairy tongue is characterized by lengthening and darkening of the papillae on the tongue.

- Causes include use of certain drugs (e.g., antibiotics), tobacco, foods, hydrogen peroxide rinses, or infectious agents; the tongue can be brushed and agents eliminated to cure this
- Phenytoin (Dilantin), certain other drugs, orthodontic braces, or plaque can cause another type of lesion called gingival hyperplasia
- Here connective tissue from the gum area expands over the teeth possibly affecting eating and appearance

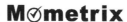

- If the irritant (for example, an essential drug) cannot be removed, surgical removal is an option
- A practice in which people put aspirin over aching root areas can cause aspirin burn in which a coarse, white lesion forms

HORMONAL CHANGE

Approximately 1 in 20 pregnant women develop pregnancy gingivitis in which the gum tissues become inflated and inflamed and occasionally tumors develop.

- These conditions should subside when hormone levels return to normal
- Another type of lesion which is often found in pregnant women, but also occurs in other women and men, is pyogenic granuloma
- This is a rapidly growing, reddened, vascular mass of granulation tissue
- It results from a combination of hormonal changes and local irritation
- Gingival swelling can also occur during the hormonal changes associated with puberty, primarily in girls
- Once hormonal balance is restored, the gingival enlargement should subside
- All of these conditions can result in bleeding at the gum unless good oral hygiene is maintained

CONGENITAL OR EARLY DEVELOPMENTAL CONDITIONS

Congenital conditions are genetically inherited states.

- There are many congenital abnormalities that may be found in the oral cavity, particularly cleft lip or palate (discussed elsewhere)
- Teeth that are unusually large or small are termed macrodontia or microdontia teeth; the latter are often associated with Down syndrome or congenital heart disease
- Amelogenesis imperfecta and dentinogenesis imperfecta are hereditary conditions affecting the enamel
- In both, the enamel is very thin and discolored (amelogenesis) or opalescent (dentinogenesis), resulting in a propensity toward caries or a wearing away of the enamel
- Certain teeth can be congenitally missing (anodontia)
- Hyperdontia is the state of having extra (supernumerary teeth)
- Teeth may be present neonatally with quick shedding after birth
- Fusion is the joining of two or more teeth:
  - There are a number of other possible fusion-like abnormalities including the following: ankylosis, the fusion of a tooth, cementum, or dentin to the alveolar bone; and gemination in which a tooth bud cannot fully divide
  - Another possible condition is twinning which is the development of two distinct teeth from one tooth bud

CLEFT LIP AND CLEFT PALATE

Both of these conditions result from the developmental failure of tissues in the oral cavity to fuse properly.

- Cleft lip occurs when maxillary processes in the head do not fuse with the medial nasal process, resulting in a notching or more pronounced indentation from the lip to nostril
- It can be unilateral (on one side) or bilateral (on both sides)

- Cleft palate occurs when the palatal shelves do not fuse with the primary palate or each other. It can be found alone or in combination with cleft lip
- There are a number of types of cleft palate depending on the fusion failure
- The least severe is cleft uvula in which only the uvula flap at the back of the soft palate fails to fuse
- Other variations include the following: bilateral cleft of the secondary palate; bilateral cleft of the lip, alveolar process, and primary palate; bilateral cleft of the lip, alveolar process, and both primary and secondary palates; and unilateral cleft lip, primary palate, and alveolar process

ORAL TORI AND EXOSTOSES

Oral tori are benign, boney extensions into the oral cavity covered with fine layers of tissue.

- Those developing from the maxillary hard palate are called torus platinus
- They occur in about 20% of adults and are usually found near the midline
- Torus mandibularis, outgrowths in canine or premolar areas of the mandible, are less common but more bothersome because food fragments can imbed there
- Both can cause tenderness during taking of oral radiographs
- They should be surgically excised if dental appliances are necessary
- Exotosis is the swelling or nodular outgrowth of lamellar bone on the facial side of the maxillary or mandibular palates. It is very similar to oral tori

DEVELOPMENTAL ABNORMALITIES

There are several possible developmental abnormalities involving the tongue.

- One of the most common is a fissured tongue in which the tongue surface is deeply grooved and sometimes asymmetrical or unevenly shaped
- A bifid tongue occurs when the sides of the front of the tongue do not fuse fully and a tip of muscle if found at the end of the tongue
- Usually both of these conditions are left untreated
- Ankyloglossia is the connection of the lingual frenum close to the tip of the tongue possibly impeding its movement and the ability to make certain sounds clearly
- It can be corrected with a simple surgical procedure that cuts the frenum
- The vast majority of individuals also have an ostensible abnormality called Fordyce's spots or granules, which are actually sebaceous oil glands close to surface epithelia in the oral mucosa

IMPROPER DIET ORAL CONDITIONS

The most common oral conditions caused by improper diet are angular cheilitis and glossitis.

- Angular cheilitis is due to a shortage of vitamin B complex
- It presents as a lesion of both the mucous membranes and skin near the corner of the mouth and changes the vertical dimension of the face
- Saliva accumulates at the corners and microorganisms can proliferate there, particularly opportunistic infections like *Candida albicans*
- The deficiency must be corrected and/or antifungal drugs must be used

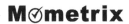

- Angular cheilitis can also develop if the person often licks the corners of the mouth or for some reason drops vertical length in the face
- Vitamin B complex deficiency is probably also the cause of glossitis or bald tongue in which the tongue is inflamed and filiform papillae are lacking

ORAL CANCER WARNING SIGNALS

Oral cancers should be suspected if the patient displays any of the following warning signals.

- One sign is a sore in the oral cavity that does not resolve within about a month
- Another symptom is protracted mouth dryness
- If there are lumps or areas of swelling anywhere in the region, including lips, oral cavity or neck, oral cancer should be considered
- White or coarse lesions on the lips or in the oral cavity can indicate malignancy
- Numbness, tenderness, or burning sensations in or near the oral cavity may be indicative of oral cancer
- Unexplained recurrent bleeding in one part of the mouth is a possible sign as well
- Lastly, if the patient has any trouble speaking, chewing, or swallowing, the clinician should investigate for the types of oral malignancy

ORAL TUMORS

There are a number of possible types of oral tumors or neoplasms some of which have the potential for malignancy.

- Papillomas are benign tumors that develop after certain viral infections, involve projections of squamous epithelial tissue, and can be surgically removed.
- Fibromas are benign areas of hyperplasia; they present as pink, even, dome-shaped lesions generally on the buccal surface.
- Lichen planus, which looks like a flattened deep red or violet bump, is condition in which the malignant potential is unclear. This is often found on the leg or ankle. When it occurs in the mouth, the buccal mucosa is usually involved and lines known as Wickham's striae may be evident. The patient usually has soreness while eating and is usually given topical steroids.

MALIGNANT OR MALIGNANT POTENTIAL

Squamous cell and basal cell carcinomas are malignant tumors of the head and neck region.

- Squamous cell carcinoma, the predominant oral cancer, involves the squamous epithelial cells. It is of great concern because it has great metastatic potential as well
- Predisposing factors include tobacco use, alcohol use, and exposure to sunlight
- Squamous cell carcinomas initially look like white plaques but later become ulcerated
- Basal cell carcinoma is the chief form of skin cancer; it is caused primarily by sunlight exposure. Here the basal cells are involved. Fortunately, this type of carcinoma rarely metastasizes and lesions can be surgically removed
- Red patches in the oral cavity that are not due to inflammation are called erythroplakia
- These patches are usually found on the floor of the mouth, the soft palate, or retro molar pad area; they are usually associated with chronic tobacco or alcohol use, and they are almost without exception malignant or premalignant

- Early erythroplakia is treated surgically and later stages with radiation and chemotherapy
- Leukoplakia, unidentifiable white, tough, hyperkeratinized patches in the mucosa that cannot be wiped off, also have malignant potential

AIDS AND HIV ORAL LESIONS

Infection with the retrovirus human immunodeficiency virus (HIV) causes an individual to have a suppressed immune system and thus susceptibility to certain opportunistic infections.

- HIV infection can eventually develop into advanced disease called acquired immunodeficiency syndrome (AIDS), which is incurable
- Good dental hygiene is imperative for AIDS patients
- They are especially vulnerable to periodontal lesions due to bacterial or fungal infections
- These patients often have *Candida albicans* fungal infections especially after chemotherapy or long-term antibiotic use
- Candida in the oral mucosa appears as thick, white lines superimposed over red, inflamed areas, particularly on the tongue or buccal regions
- It should be treated with antifungals such as Nystatin
- HIV positive individuals may also have similar hairy leukoplakia or white patterns near the edges of the tongue
- The vascular malignancy Kaposi's sarcoma is particularly associated with AIDS
- It presents as scattered bluish-purple lesions on the palate and in other areas such as the face and arms
- Eventually these lesions can hemorrhage and low-dose radiation and/or chemotherapy are indicated

ORAL CAVITY DISORDERS

Disorders of the oral cavity include:

- One of the most common miscellaneous disorders is geographic tongue in which there are smooth red patches usually bounded by yellow or white edges on the back and sides of the tongue. In addition, filiform papillae (hairy extensions) are missing. Geographic tongue does not hurt and requires no intervention.
- An infectious disorder called acute necrotizing ulcerative gingivitis (ANUG) often occurs in teenagers and young adults. In addition to infection, ANUG is characterized by oral cavity pain, bleeding, and a foul odor. The affected area must be cleansed, dead and infected tissue removed. Antibiotics and hot water rinses are indicated.
- Another possible condition is development of a mucocele or bump inside the upper lip. This is actually the closing off of a salivary duct after trauma such as biting the lip; sometimes the salivary gland needs to be opened and the accumulated fluid extracted.
- Other miscellaneous disorders include varix, weakened and distended blood vessels in the cavity, and drooping features as a consequence of Bell's palsy, which is a temporary paralysis of the facial muscles on one side.

ANOREXIA NERVOSA OR BULIMIA

These are two eating disorders. Anorexia nervosa is characterized by unrealistic fears and weight loss of at least 15% while bulimia is distinguished by periods of uncontrollable eating followed by induced vomiting. Along with other health threats, both can affect the appearance of the oral cavity.

- In particular, the vomiting accompanying bulimia can causes changes in the oral cavity
- Typically, the lingual surfaces of the front teeth lose calcium and the enamel wears away

31

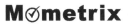

- The occlusal faces of back teeth also erode
- If the patient has had restorative work done, the fillings begin to fail
- These patients tend to have quite a few cavities and enlarged parotid glands
- Good oral hygiene is imperative, particularly after vomiting, and toothpaste for sensitive teeth is recommended

Charting

UNIVERSAL AND PALMER (QUADRANT) NUMBERING SYSTEMS

Orientation of the chart is traditionally "patient's view", i.e. patient's right corresponds to notation-chart right:

Universal numbering system table															
Permanent Teeth															
upper left								upper right							
16	15	14	13	12	11	10	9	8	7	6	5	4	3	2	1
17	18	19	20	21	22	23	24	25	26	27	28	29	30	31	32
lower left								lower right							
Deciduous teeth (baby teeth)															
upper left								upper right							
		J	I	H	G	F		E	D	C	B	A			
		K	L	M	N	O		P	Q	R	S	T			
lower left								lower right							
Alternate system for Deciduous teeth															
upper left								upper right							
		10d	9d	8d	7d		6d	5d	4d	3d	2d	1d			
		11d	12d	13d	14d		15d	16d	17d	18d	19d	20d			
lower left								lower right							

PALMER NOTATION OF PERMANENT TEETH

Orientation of the chart is traditionally "dentist's view", i.e. patient's right corresponds to notation chart left. The designations "left" and "right" on the chart, however, nonetheless correspond to the patient's left and right, respectively:

Palmer notation															
Permanent Teeth															
upper right								upper left							
8⌋	7⌋	6⌋	5⌋	4⌋	3⌋	2⌋	1⌋	L1	L2	L3	L4	L5	L6	L7	L8
8⌐	7⌐	6⌐	5⌐	4⌐	3⌐	2⌐	1⌐	Γ1	Γ2	Γ3	Γ4	Γ5	Γ6	Γ7	Γ8
lower right								lower left							
Deciduous teeth (baby teeth)															
upper right								upper left							
		E⌋	D⌋	C⌋	B⌋	A⌋		LA	LB	LC	LD	LE			
		E⌐	D⌐	C⌐	B⌐	A⌐		ΓA	ΓB	ΓC	ΓD	ΓE			
lower right								lower left							

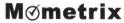

CLASSIFICATIONS OF DENTAL CAVITIES

Dental cavities or caries are classified from Class I to Class VI based on the teeth and surfaces in which they are formed. Classes I to V was described by a pioneer in the field of dentistry, G. V. Black, and Class VI was included later. The classifications are as follows:

- Class I - developmental caries in pits and fissures, including occlusal surfaces of back teeth, buccal or lingual pits on molars, and lingual pits on maxillary incisors, usually filled with tooth-colored composite resins
- Class II - cavities on proximal surfaces of premolars or molars, restored with tooth-colored resins, silver amalgam, or sometimes gold or porcelain
- Class III - cavities on interproximal surfaces of incisors or canines, filled with composite resins
- Class IV - similar to Class III except incisal edge is also involved, restored with composites and if considerable decay, porcelain crowns as well
- Class V - caries only near the gum line on either facial or lingual surface, composites usually used for front teeth, silver amalgam possible for posterior teeth
- Class VI - cavities on occlusal or incisal surfaces formed by wearing away, varied restoration materials

CHARTING CARIES OR CAVITIES

Cavities are charted in terms of whether they involve single, two, or three or more surfaces that have been or need to be restored.

- A simple cavity restoration involves only a single surface
- Simple cavity restorations are described by a letter standing for the surface involved as follows: I (incisal), M (mesial), D (distal), B (buccal), O (occlusal), or F (facial)
- Compound or two-surface restorations use a combination of two letters that illustrate the two facades involved
- Typical compound cavity restorations would be described as OB (occlusobuccal), MO (mesio-occlusal), MI (mesio-incisal), DO (disto-occlusal), DI (disto-incisal), DL (disto-lingual), or LI (lingual-incisal)
- Complex cavity restorations are those that involve at least three surfaces, and the abbreviations for them incorporate all facades involved, for example MOD for mesio-occluso-distal

BASIC CHARTING TERMS

Some basic charting terms that are descriptive include the following:

- Abscess - a limited infected area usually filled with pus
- Diastema - the gap between two teeth, usually used to describe that between maxillary central incisors
- Drifting - movement of tooth position to occupy spaces formed by removal of another, also called overeruption
- Incipient - areas of developing decay where enamel is still intact, appearance is chalky due to initiation of decalcification
- Mobility - movement of a tooth within the socket generally as a result of trauma or periodontal disease, usually quantified in millimeters

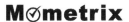

- Periodontal pocket - excessive space in sulcus of gum due to periodontal disease (usually more than 3 mm), similarly quantified
- Overhang - presence of too much restorative material

DENTAL WORK DONE

Basic charting terms referring to actual dental work done or suggested include the following:

- Bridge - a prosthesis that replaces missing teeth, usually held in place on the attaching sides (abutments) or sometimes just one side (a cantilever bridge); middle area is termed the pontic
- Crown - custom-made permanent or manufactured temporary tops that are attached to teeth; available in a variety of materials and combinations including gold, porcelain, stainless steel and plastic; generally cover either the full or ¾ of the tooth
- Denture - a complete (full arch) or partial set of artificial teeth generally attached to a plate
- Restoration - materials (silver amalgams, composite resins, and gold) used to fill cavities or otherwise replace missing tooth structure
- Root canal - a procedure in which the pulp is taken out and replaced with a filling material
- Sealant - a resin that is employed to seal pits and fissures in the tooth enamel to deter decay
- Veneer - a thin material bonded only to the facial aspect of the tooth

TYPICAL CHARTING SYMBOLS

Dental work that needs to be done is generally indicated in red on a chart while work that has already been done is shown in blue.

- Missing teeth are indicated by an "X" through the tooth or teeth on the chart
- If all teeth in an arch are missing, that arch is indicated by encircling it and placing an "X" over it
- Supernumerary or extra teeth are drawn in on the chart
- Drifting or over-erupted teeth are shown by arrows in the direction of the drift
- Teeth that are currently or have been impacted or unerupted are circled
- Teeth requiring extraction generally have a red slash through them
- Diastema is indicated by two vertical lines at the gap
- Tooth rotation is shown with a directional arrow on the side and mobility with two small lines
- Areas of tooth or root fracture are shown as jagged lines
- Teeth that need or have completed root canals are indicated with vertical lines in red or blue respectively
- Gingival recession or furcation involvement is shown with wavy lines and dots
- An abscess is shown with a small red circle in the area near the root
- Arrows between roots are indicative of periodontal pockets
- Caries are indicated in red or blue, depending on whether or not they have been restored. The surfaces that are affected are either filled in or encircled with the appropriate color
- Amalgam restorations are usually shown by both outlining and filling in and composites with outlining
- Recurrent decay of previously restored teeth is indicated by outlining the existing restoration in red
- For enamel sealants that have been used to deter decay, an "S" is placed over the area
- Temporary restorations are generally indicated with blue circles

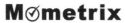

- For crowns, diagonal lines are drawn across the whole area involved if gold, or encircled if porcelain
- For fixed bridges, an "X" is drawn through the root(s) of missing teeth and the area for the bridge is either outlined (porcelain) or indicated by diagonal lines (gold)
- A Maryland bridge, which has wings on the pontic, shows them with curves
- Veneers are indicated by outlining
- For dentures, "X"s are placed over all involved root areas and the corresponding crown areas are shown by either a large circle (full) or dotted lines (partial)

PERIODONTAL DISEASES

Periodontal diseases involve the periodontium, the tissue that surrounds and holds up the teeth.

- They can lead to tooth loss through lack of support
- Most periodontal disease starts as inflammation resulting from the buildup of plaque or bacterial colonies sticking to teeth or areas of the gingivae
- Mineralized plaque on teeth is called dental calculus, and caries can develop from plaque when sugars are converted into acids by the bacteria
- Periodontal disease can also result from hormonal disturbances or other oral problems
- Risk factors include diabetes, poor oral hygiene, osteoporosis, stress, certain medications, HIV/AIDS, irritation from dental appliances, and malocclusion
- One type of periodontal disease involves the gums or gingivae; the presence of inflamed and possibly bleeding gums is referred to as gingivitis
- If the bacterial infection spreads to the underlying supporting alveolar bone, periodontitis results

PERIODONTITIS CLASSIFICATION SCHEME

In addition to the gingival and alveolar bone, other structures in the periodontium may be involved including the epithelial attachment, the periodontal ligaments in contact with the root and alveolar bone, and the cementum or bony tissue covering the roots.

- Periodontal disease classification is related to involvement of all of these structures, how aggressive the disease is, whether or not necrosis has occurred, and the size of the sulcus or space dividing the tooth and free gingival
- Class I or chronic periodontitis is characterized inflammation of the area, destruction of the periodontal ligament, bone damage, and tooth mobility; it is subdivided into slight, moderate and severe categories based on depth of pockets of detachment, degree of bone loss, and tooth mobility
- For molars, furcation involvement is considered
- Class II or aggressive periodontitis is early-onset and involves rapidly progressing destruction of tissue and clinical signs of inflammation
- It can occur as prepubertal periodontitis, beginning sometime before the eruption of the primary teeth and puberty (usually localized), or as juvenile periodontitis (either localized or systemic)
- Class III or necrotizing periodontal disease is ulcerative tissue death

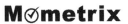

CHARTING PERIODONTAL CONDITIONS OR PRECURSORS

Excessive dental plaque, which can lead to periodontal disease, is indicated on the chart by a squiggly line above the tooth. On the chart, periodontal pockets are usually indicated with an arrow and number indicating depths. A true periodontal chart usually enumerates the periodontal pocket depth for each tooth on both the facial and lingual sides.

- Tooth mobility is classified as normal (0), slight (1), moderate (2) or severe (3)
- Areas of exudate or pus are noted
- The gingival recession is also shown by drawing a dotted or colored line along the gum line, which visualizes the degree to which each root is exposed
- Furcation involvement for the molar area is noted

PERIODONTAL EXAMINATION ELEMENTS

A periodontal examination has several components beyond histories.

- Good radiographs can show evidence of periodontal disease
- Examination of the teeth includes assessment of tooth mobility with two instruments, inspection of the gingivae and supporting structures, and examination of any periodontal pockets with a probe
- Periodontal probes, standardized in millimeters, are used to measure depths of six surfaces, the facial, lingual, distofacial, distolingual, semiofficial, and mesiolingual; the deepest is usually logged by the dental assistant
- As discussed elsewhere, a periodontal chart is completed, which includes pocket depths, furcations, mobility, exudates, and gingival recession
- The dentist typically also uses explorers to find calculus and assess the root, straight or curved scalers to get rid of supragingival calculus, and less blunt curettes to remove subgingival calculus

NORMAL OCCLUSION AND FACIAL PROFILES

Occlusion is the relationship between upper and lower teeth when the mouth is closed.

- In normal occlusion, teeth in both dental arches are in maximum contact without rotation or nonstandard spacing
- The front teeth in the maxillary arch overlap the incisal edge of those in the mandible slightly by about 2 millimeters
- The maxillary posterior teeth are positioned one cusp further back than the mandibular posterior ones
- Lastly, the mesial buccal cusp of the first permanent molar in the upper arch is in contact with the buccal groove of the first molar in the mandible
- Normal occlusion should give a mesognathic facial profile, a fairly straight line between jaws with only a slight projection of the mandible relative to the upper part of the face

MALOCCLUSION AND ANGLE'S CLASSIFICATIONS

Malocclusion is any divergence from normal occlusion.

- Angle's classifications are used most often to describe three basic types of malocclusion
- The first is neutroclusion (Class I) in which occlusion is essentially normal except that individual or groups of teeth are out of position; the facial profile is still mesognathic
- The next is distoclusion (Class II) in which the buccal groove of the mandibular first permanent molar is behind the mesiobuccal cusp of the corresponding maxillary molar

- Distoclusion can be Division 1 or 2 due to either outward protrusion of the maxillary teeth or backward sloping of the mandibular teeth
- Both produce a retrognathic facial profile where one or both jaws are recessed
- The last classification of malocclusion is mesioclusion (Class III) in which the buccal groove of the mandibular first permanent molar is mesial to the mesiobuccal cusp of the corresponding maxillary molar
- Here the facial profile is prognathic meaning the jaws project beyond the upper part of the face

MALOCCLUSION CAUSES

Malocclusion is caused by one of three types of factors. Inherited genetic factors can contribute to formation of extra or supernumerary teeth, missing teeth, atypical relationships between the jaws or between teeth and the jaw, and deviations such as cleft palate.

- Exposure to certain systemic diseases or nutritional deficiencies during the formative years can interrupt the normal developmental pattern of dentition
- Particular habits or localized trauma can produce malocclusion
- These include breathing by mouth, thumb or tongue sucking, thrusting of the tongue, nail biting, and bruxism
- Bruxism is the unconscious grinding of teeth during sleep or stressful situations

MALPOSITIONS

Individual teeth can exhibit the following variations and contribute to malocclusion.

- Teeth that are mesial, distal, or lingual to their normal position are examples of mesioversion, distoversion, and linguoversion respectively
- Torsiversion is the rotation or turning of a tooth from the expected position
- Buccoversion or labioversion is the inclination of a tooth toward the cheek or lip
- If the crown of an individual tooth is outside the normal line of occlusion, it exhibits either supraversion (above) or infraversion (below)
- A tooth may appear in the wrong position or order of the dental arch, a variation called transversion or transposition

OVERBITE AND AN OVERJET

These are two types of malpositions between groups of teeth that result in malocclusion. Both are teeth overlaps.

- An overbite is a greater than normal vertical overlap between anterior maxillary and mandibular teeth. An overbite occurs when the upper incisors extend over more than one-third of the front teeth in the mandible
- An overjet is horizontal overlap. Here there is an unusually large horizontal distance between the outer surface of the anterior mandibular teeth and the inner face of the maxillary anterior teeth
- A person can also have an underjet in which the front teeth in the mandible project significantly in front of the maxillary anterior teeth

CROSSBITES

A cross-bite is an atypical relationship between single or groups of teeth in one dental arch relative to the other.

- With a cross-bite involving anterior teeth, the incisors in the maxilla are lingual to the opposing ones in the mandible
- Posterior cross-bite presents similarly with maxillary back teeth closer to the tongue than the mandibular teeth, the opposite of that expected with a normal bite
- There can also be an edge-edge bite in which the incisal surfaces of teeth in both arches converge, an end-to-end bite between posterior teeth whose cusps meet, or an open bite in which there is a lack of occlusion between the mandibular and maxillary teeth
- Overbites and overjets are discussed elsewhere

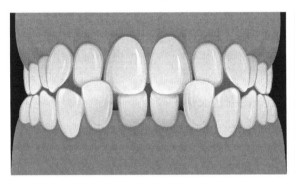 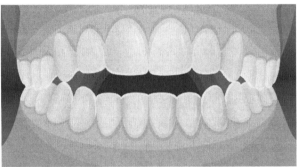

FACE LANDMARKS

The landmarks of the face and oral cavity are observed during examination for abnormalities.

- Beginning in the nasal area, the first facial landmark is the outside edge or ala of the nose
- Extending from there to the corner of the mouth is the naso-labial groove
- Another distinguishing feature of the face is the philtrum, the hollow in-between the bottom of the nose and the center of the upper lip
- The lip area is characterized by four facial landmarks:
  - (1) the vermillion zone, the entire reddish part of the lips
  - (2) the vermillion border surrounding it
  - (3) the tubercle of the lip, the slight protrusion in the center of the upper lip
  - (4) the labial commissures, the corners of the mouth

- The lip vermillion zone is highly vascularized which contributes to its color
- The final facial landmark is the labio-mental groove, a horizontal depression in the middle between the lip and chin

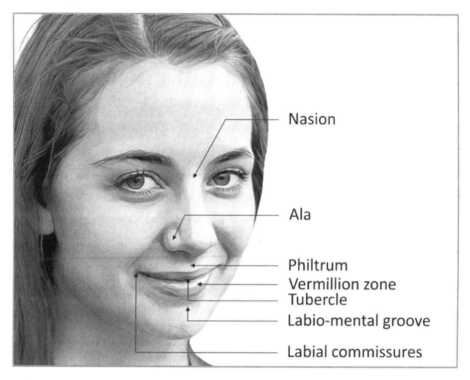

ORAL CAVITY LANDMARKS

The oral cavity is characterized by the oral vestibule or mucobuccal fold, the pouch created where the soft cheek tissue and gums come together. Its continuous border is the vestibule fornix. There are several characteristic mucosae or moist linings in the oral cavity. These include the following:

- the labial mucosa on the inside of the lips
- the buccal mucosa on the interior of the cheeks
- the looser, redder alveolar mucosa encasing the alveolar bone shoring up the teeth

On the labial mucosa near the corners of the mouth are other landmarks called Fordyce's spots, minute yellow glands.

- The buccal mucosa contains two characteristic features, an elevated white line at the level where teeth come together called the linea alba and a piece of skin across from the maxillary second molar known as the parotid papilla
- Another landmark is the gingiva or pink, fibrous tissue near the teeth
- The oral cavity also should have two types of frena (plural of frenum) or restraining folds of tissue, the labial frena (the major ones between the central incisors in either jaw) and the buccal frena

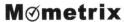

ORAL CAVITY PALATE PORTION

The palate is the roof of the mouth interior to the maxillary teeth.

- The front or hard palate is comprised of a bony plate enveloped with pink keratinized tissue, and the back or soft palate is made of muscle
- Landmarks on the hard palate are the incisive papilla (an elevated area behind the top central incisors); and ridges that run either down the center toward the back, a single palatine raphe, or horizontally across the hard palate posterior to the incisive papilla, the palatine rugae
- There may also be a torus palatinus or bone protuberance in the center of the palate
- In the soft palate area, there is a uvula or outcrop of tissue at the back of it and anterior tonsillar pillars that arch toward the tongue
- Extending behind the soft palate into the oropharynx area are the posterior tonsillar pillars
- The palatine tonsils are located between these two arches or pillars
- At the rear of the oral cavity is the entrance to the pharynx, the fauces

TONGUE AND FLOOR OF THE MOUTH

The dorsal or top side of the tongue is distinguished by the presence of several types of papilla or projections in the anterior two thirds bearing the taste buds, a groove called the median sulcus dividing the front portion in half, and another groove in the back called the sulcus terminalis.

- The types of papilla and their locations should be large circumvallate papillae in front of the sulcus terminalis, hair-like protrusions called filiform papillae further forward, redder fungiform papillae near the front part, and tissue creases on the sides termed foliate papillae
- The ventral or under side of the tongue is distinguished by a central line of tissue termed the lingual frenum, which continues into the floor of the mouth
- There are lingual veins to either side and tissue creases called fimbriated folds on the sides
- At the point of attachment of the lingual frenum to the floor of the mouth, there are tissue folds called sublingual caruncles
- Sublingual folds branch from there and there is a sublingual sulcus close to the dental arch

SALIVARY GLANDS

Salivary glands secrete saliva into the oral cavity.

- Saliva is used to moisten food and tissues in the oral space, facilitate chewing and ingestion, aid digestion of starches, and normalize water balance
- It is a transparent liquid usually of slightly alkaline pH and containing water, mucin protein, organic salts, and an enzyme called ptyalin
- Saliva is primarily secreted from three pairs of salivary glands and adjoining ducts that drain the saliva into the mouth:
  - The parotid glands are located ahead of the ear; their parotid or Stensen's ducts empty into the area around the maxillary second molars
  - The submandibular glands are located in the rear of the mandible; their Warton's ducts drain into the sublingual caruncles
  - The sublingual glands are positioned on the floor of the mouth and can empty either right into the mouth via the ducts of Rivinus or indirectly via the ducts of Bartholin into the sublingual caruncles

41

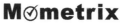

MAXILLA AND PALATE

The maxilla or upper jaw is the biggest facial bone encompassing the region from the eye sockets and nasal cavities to form the roof of the oral cavity.

- It is actually two segments of bone held together in the middle by the median suture
- The maxilla develops from four bone outgrowths or processes, the frontal, zygomatic, alveolar, and palatine
- There are openings called the infraorbital foramen beneath the eye sockets, sizeable openings called the maxillary sinuses near the roots of the top molars, and a rounded area in the back called the maxillary tuberosity
- The palatine bones are fused at the midline by the palatine suture with a connection to the nasopalatine nerve near the front called the incisive foramen
- There should also be a horizontally located transverse palatine suture near the back of the hard palate
- Posterior to it on each side are three other openings, one greater palatine foramen and two lesser palatine foramina

MANDIBLE

The only facial bone that can move is the lower jaw or mandible.

- Basically, the mandible is curved in front in a horizontal plane (following the dental arch) and has vertical wings at the back called rami
- The rami are capped by two projections, the condyloid process in the back (which connects to the temporal bone to form the temporomandibular joint) and the sharper coronoid process anterior to it
- From the ramus area proceeding forward, are the mandibular and mental foramens on the outside and the lingual foramen on the tongue side plus various characteristic ridges
- The front of the mandible is distinguished by a depression in the center called the symphysis
- This is where the bones meet
- The apex of the chin is the mental protuberance

TEMPOROMANDIBULAR JOINT

The temporomandibular joint (TMJ) is a junction formed by the glenoid fossa and articular eminence of the temporal bone and the condyloid process of the mandible.

- The temporal bones on either side of the face are cranial bones
- The joint is immersed in synovial fluid, and the bones are enclosed by cartilage and supported by a number of ligaments
- The condyloid process or condyle is padded with fibrous connective tissue called the articular disc or meniscus
- When the mouth is closed, the meniscus is in close contact (separated by cavities bathed in synovial fluid) with the glenoid fossa of the temporal bone and the articular eminence further forward
- As the mouth opens, normally initially a hinge motion develops as the condyles and discs move forward

- Then, the condyles and discs move further forward as the mouth opens more in a forward gliding joint movement
- If the meniscus gets trapped or dislocated, TMJ disease can occur usually manifesting as a characteristic clicking noise

CRANIUM AND FACE

Cranial bones enclose and protect the brain. The bones of the face are as follows:

- 2 temporal bones at the lower sides and base of the skull
- a frontal bone in the forehead area
- 2 parietal bones on the top and upper sides of the head
- the occipital bone at the rear and base of the skull
- the sphenoid bone in front of the temporal area
- ethmoid bones, creating part of the nose, eye sockets, and floor of the cranium

There are also various processes and sinuses. There are 8 types of facial bones.

- there are a set of nasal bones constituting the bridge of the nose
- one vomer bone inside forming part of the nasal septum separating the two cavities
- inferior nasal conchae inside the cavity
- there are two lacrimal bones that are part of the orbit of the eye
- Zygomatic bones create the cheeks and are also part of the maxilla or upper jaw
- Two maxillae
- the set of palatine
- the mandible bones

TMJ DYSFUNCTION

Temporomandibular joint (TMJ) dysfunction is the lack of coordination of the structures associated with the TMJ.

- It can present as pain near the ear often extending into the face, soreness in the muscles involved with chewing, popping or clicking noises upon opening or closing the mouth, other sounds like crepitus (crackling) or tinnitus (ringing), headache or neck pain, and lack of ability to adequately open the mouth (trismus) or move the lower jaw
- Usually, diagnosis of TMJ dysfunction or disease is made based on a combination of medical and dental history, physical examination, evaluation by tomographic radiography or magnetic resonance imaging, and casts of the teeth to replicate the movements of the jaws
- In particular, the history normally includes questioning about grinding or clamping of the teeth, bite issues, injuries or diseases that may affect TMJ function, and stress
- The clinician examines the area by palpation, takes note of characteristic sounds while the jaw is opened and closed, and also quantifies how wide the person can open his or her mouth

TREATMENT FOR TMJ DYSFUNCTION

Some treatment options for TMJ dysfunction are relatively minor, such as stress management, rotating heat and cold application, resting the jaw, or use of various medications.

- The types of medications used include pain relievers, such as nonsteroidal anti-inflammatory agents (NSAIDs), muscle relaxants, antibiotics, and drugs that affect the nervous system (e.g., mood enhancers or anti-anxiety drugs)

- Certain practices like physical therapy or massage are often helpful
- There are also a number of more extreme treatments for TMJ disease
- Steroids may be injected into the intra-articular area
- There are occlusal splints that can be constructed to alleviate spasms or pressure
- Often the disorder is treated with orthodontia and other restoration
- There are several types of surgery that can be used, including arthroscopic removal of adhesions coupled with insertion of anti-inflammatory agents or open joint surgery in which the joints are actually reconstructed

Diagnostic Data

RADIOGRAPHY PROCEDURES

The dental assistant should make sure the dental chair is covered with plastic or another type of barrier.

- Any parts of the radiographic equipment or room that will be touched should also be wrapped with plastic
- He or she should also set up all required instruments, films, and paraphernalia (e.g., cotton rolls) that might be needed
- It is important to protect the patient and the technician against radiation exposure
- The assistant should wear gloves, protective eyeglasses, and a mask
- The patient should remove all metal objects from the facial area and wear a lead apron with a thyroid collar during the exposure
- Then, the tubehead of the x-ray machine can be brought in and the technician can proceed with taking the photographs
- Once each radiograph is taken, the film is removed, saliva is wiped off, and the film is put in a paper cup or on a special barrier
- After the complete set of films is taken, the assistant can take off the patient's lead apron either by removing his or her gloves or wearing an overglove
- Films are then dispatched to processing. Infection control procedures should be followed for cleanup

INTRAORAL RADIOGRAPHS

There are three main types of intraoral radiographs.

- The first type, a periapical radiographs, is generally unnecessary in the orthodontic context.
  - o Periapical radiographs look at the entire tooth and the area around it to appraise general tooth, bone and tissue health, tooth development, and presence of disease
- The second type is the bite-wing radiograph of front teeth
  - o Bite-wing or interproximal radiographs generally show crowns, crest of the alveolar bone, and interproximal gaps in both arches
  - o Their primary purposes are detection of cavities, bad restorations, and calculus and the assessment of the crestal area
- Occlusal radiographs attempt to look at one of the dental arches in its entirety and picture the occlusal surfaces

INTRAORAL RADIOGRAPHS

There are two methods that can be used for taking intraoral radiographs, either the bisecting technique or the paralleling technique.

- The bisecting technique is older and less often used today
- All intraoral radiographs can be taken using the bisecting method
- The guiding principle of the technique is that the central x-ray should be aimed perpendicular to an imaginary line that bisects the angle between the longitudinal axis of the tooth and the plane of the dental film
- The path of the central ray is the vertical angulation

- The head is positioned more upright for maxillary exposures and tilted back for mandibular ones as the goal is to have occlusal surfaces photographed parallel to the floor
- The film to be exposed is positioned near the lingual surface without much extending above the occlusal surface
- There are tables that suggest vertical angulation for a particular x-ray tubehead
- Maxillary shots have positive vertical angulation and mandibular exposures have slightly negative vertical angulation
- The other parameter, horizontal angulation or height of the x-ray tube relative to the floor, is set through directing the beam at interproximal spaces

PARALLELING TECHNIQUE PRINCIPLES

The paralleling technique is more common today than the bisecting method.

- The paralleling technique dictates that the film packet must be parallel to the longitudinal axis of the teeth being photographed and the central x-ray beam must be aimed perpendicular to both packet and long axis
- In order to accomplish this, intraoral radiographs by the paralleling method generally require more centrally located film packets and use of film holders
- Film holders (Snap-a-Ray, Rinn XCP, etc.) are used with the holder and film parallel to the longitudinal axis of the teeth; the dot on the film should be toward the area being photographed and usually peaks of the teeth are about 1/8 inch from the top of the film
- The film holders usually have a positioning ring that aids the technician with directing the x-ray beam
- Generally, if the cone of the x-ray equipment is aimed even with the positioning ring, correct vertical and horizontal angulation as well as complete covering of the film should be guaranteed

BITE-WING SERIES

Usually, a bite-wing series of radiographs covers the premolar and molar areas, although bite-wings can be taken of anterior teeth.

- They are routinely taken during dental examinations either as components of a full-mouth survey or once or twice a year alone
- Bite-wings are usually done with horizontal positioning using four No. 2 (or sometimes No. 3) films for adults and usually No. 0 or 1 (but sometimes No. 2) size films for children
- Vertical bite-wing radiographs are increasingly being solicited, especially by periodontists
- Vertical positioning illustrates the root area better and can pick up root caries, periodontal gaps, and bone deficiencies
- With a special holding device, vertical bite-wings can be taken in any area
- Vertical and horizontal angulation principles are the same for either type of positioning
- X-ray beams should be aimed interproximally so that teeth do not overlap on the radiograph
- If used as part of full-mouth radiographic survey in an adult, generally 4 bite-wing and 14 periapical radiographs are taken

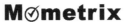

MAXILLARY INCISORS AND CUSPIDS POSITIONING

For all films, the film is inserted into the slot on the bite-block and the ring on the rod is fine-tuned so that it covers the entire film.

- Then, the tubehead is brought into the area of exposure and the film is positioned before exposure
- For maxillary incisors, the film and its holder are inclined downward and placed rather centrally away from the lingual surfaces of the teeth being photographed
- The individual closes his or her mouth and bites down
- The positioning ring is then pushed close to the person's face
- The x-ray machine cone is positioned approximately one-half inch from the ring and parallel to the attached metal rod in order to establish a perpendicular relationship between the central x-ray and film
- The incisal edge abuts directly onto the flat part of the bite-block
- For adults, a No. 2 size film is generally used to cover all maxillary central and lateral incisors
- Positioning for taking radiographs of maxillary cuspids is similarly tilted and positioned with the central x-ray aimed at the center of the cuspid

MAXILLARY PREMOLARS AND MOLARS POSITIONING

As with maxillary incisors and cuspids, the film and holder are tilted downward and placed away from the lingual side of the tooth toward the center for radiographs of maxillary premolars and molars.

- For maxillary premolars, the front edge of the film is positioned near the middle of the cuspid and the bite-block is centered on the premolars
- The cone of the tubehead should be placed such that the central ray is delivered right to the area where the first and second premolars meet
- Films and holders are slanted a little more horizontally for maxillary molar radiographs such that the film is parallel to the lingual surface of the molars
- The focal point of the bite-block is on the second molar

INCISORS AND CUSPIDS POSITIONING

For radiographs of portions of the mandibular arch, the cone and film/holder assembly are always tilted slightly upwards relative to the ground.

- The film holder and film rest on the floor of the mouth in back of and away from the lingual surface for shots of the mandibular incisors
- The patient may need to reposition the tongue in order to place the film far enough back
- The bite-block is positioned with the incisors in the center and the central ray is aimed between the central incisors
- Both central and lateral sets of mandibular incisors are generally covered
- For exposures of mandibular cuspids, the major difference is that the film is centered on the cuspid

47

MANDIBULAR PREMOLARS AND MOLARS POSITIONING

As with other shots of the mandible, the film and its holder should be tilted slightly upwards and between the lingual side of the tooth and the tongue for both premolars and molars.

- For mandibular premolars, the front edge of the film is placed in the middle of the cuspid to ensure exposure of both premolars
- There is a parallel relationship between film, teeth and the tip of the cone
- For radiographs of the mandibular molars, the bite-block should be centered over the second molar
- Some special positioning tactics such as manually placing the person's cheek over the bite-block, repositioning the tongue toward the middle of the mouth, or holding the bite-block while the individual bites down may be needed

PREMOLAR BITE-WING POSITIONING

Bite-wing radiographs require use of a positioning apparatus comprised of a holder, an indicator rod, and a positioning ring. Alternatively, an adhesive-backed tab might be used.

- In either case, the film should be placed in the middle of the bite-wing holder with the smooth side facing the positioning ring
- For premolar bite-wing radiographs, the side edges of the film should be placed at approximately the middle of the cuspid and the second molars
- If a tab is used, it is positioned near the lingual surface and behind the mandibular premolars
- With a positioning device, the bite-wing holder is put in the mouth parallel to and away from the lingual surface of the premolars
- The vertical angulation is neutral or 0°, and the horizontal angulation is set such that the central beam is aimed where the maxillary and mandibular premolars meet

MOLAR BITE-WING RADIOGRAPHS POSITIONING

Molar bite-wing radiographs are taken using tabs or positioning devices just as with premolar bite-wings.

- The film is sited with the front edge within the distal portion of the second premolar extending posteriorly past the third molar
- The film is positioned away from the lingual surfaces of the molars
- This usually requires repositioning of the tongue away from these surfaces
- Just as with premolar bite-wings, the vertical angulation is 0° to maintain a perpendicular relationship between film and x-ray beam, and the horizontal angulation is set to direct the x-ray beam at the plane between the first and second molars of each dental arch with the mouth closed

OCCLUSAL RADIOGRAPHS

Occlusal radiographs are taken using large films.

- The patient bites down on these films
- Occlusal radiographs are useful for identifying many unusual conditions as they cover a large portion of the dental arch
- Occlusal radiographs are exposed by using one of two methods, either the topographic technique or the cross-section technique
- The topographic technique utilizes the tenets of bisecting (not parallelism)

48

- Maxillary views are taken by positioning the individual with the maxillary arch parallel to the floor
- The patient bites down on the film with about 2mm of film outside the mouth
- The cone is directed from above with a vertical angulation of between +65° to +75° over the bridge of the nose, making sure the incisors are included
- A mandibular view is taken with the person's head inclined backwards, a vertical angulation in the range of -40° to -55°, and the cone aimed from below toward the tip of the chin

CROSS-SECTION TECHNIQUE

In addition to the topographic method, occlusal radiographs can also be exposed using the cross-section technique.

- The cross-section technique also uses bisecting principles
- For both views, the central x-ray is directed at a 90° angle perpendicular to the film placement
- This means that for the maxillary view, the person's head is inclined slightly backward and the cone is directed over the bridge of the nose, but in this case it is positioned over the top of the patient's head
- Similarly for the mandibular view, the person is lying with the head tilted much further back and the cone is placed under the chin with the central ray directed perpendicular to the film

PEDIATRIC RADIOGRAPHS

Children have hypersensitive oral mucosa.

- They must be examined cautiously
- Radiographic documentation of the oral cavity must be altered to keep radiation exposure to a minimum (by reducing exposure time or taking as few radiographs as possible), reduce time involved, and minimize apprehension and discomfort
- Generally, much smaller films, either size No. 0 or1, are used for all exposures except occlusal views (No. 2)
- Front films are usually taken first, and the paralleling technique is usually employed
- A full-mouth pediatric survey for a young child typically includes two bite-wings and some combination of periapical and/or occlusal radiographs. For example, maxillary and mandibular occlusals, two bite-wings, and four periapicals might be taken

DECIDUOUS AND PERMANENT TEETH RADIOGRAPHS

In many cases, the techniques for taking radiographs of pediatric deciduous or primary teeth vary little from those used with permanent teeth.

- For example, occlusal films of the maxillary and mandibular arches are taken essentially as they are for adults
- Deciduous bite-wing radiographs differ in that the film is placed to include the first and second molars with the front edge in the center of the cuspid
- The positioning for maxillary deciduous molars using a film holder is also similar except that in this case placing the front edge of the film in the center of the cuspid ensures that the first and second deciduous molars are covered
- The central ray should be focused through the meeting point of the two molars
- Placement is similar for the mandibular deciduous molars with the usual positioning between the tongue and mandibular arch

PANORAMIC RADIOGRAPHY

Extraoral radiographs are utilized to look at larger areas of the head all at once.

- The most commonly used techniques are panoramic and cephalometric radiography
- Panoramic radiography is very useful for assessment of the complete dentition, malocclusion, other structures such as alveolar bone and sinuses, the temporomandibular joint area, and a variety of conditions
- The basic principle of panoramic radiography is the oppositional rotation of a film cassette and an x-ray head to give a panoramic view of the head
- Special panoramic x-ray machines are used
- A large extraoral film is placed in the cassette using safelight procedures sandwiched between two intensifying screens embedded with phosphors that emit light when hit by x-rays
- Both hard and soft cassettes are available
- The type of film used is dependent on the phosphors in the intensifying screen, either fast rare-earth phosphors that emit green light or slower blue light phosphors
- The patient dons a lead apron without a thyroid collar as the x-ray beam is aimed upward with minimal thyroid exposure
- They must remain still during exposure and remove all potential artifacts

CEPHALOMETRIC RADIOGRAPHY

Cephalometric radiography is used to examine the overall skeletal structure and soft tissues of the patient's head.

- It generally covers a larger view (typically the entire head) than a panoramic radiograph and is utilized primarily by orthodontists for planning purposes
- A cephalometric radiography device usually consists of a contrivance that holds the head (a cephalostat), a large cassette holder, and an x-ray tubehead
- Patients are always positioned such that the Frankfort plane, the line between the tragus of the ear and the floor of the orbit of the eye, is parallel to the ground, and the x-ray beam is aimed at a 90° angle to the cassette
- The patient is either standing or seated
- Lateral views are taken by having the person place the side of his or her head against the cassette with the midsagittal or dividing plane parallel to it. If a cephalostat is unavailable, the seated patient can hold the cassette
- In either case, the tubehead is placed on the other side

RADIOPAQUE AND RADIOLUCENT

Radiographs are created by exposing areas of the body to low levels of a type of electromagnetic energy called x-rays and capturing the image on film.

- Structures that are dense, such as intact teeth, either completely block or only absorb part of the x-ray beam and are termed radiopaque
- On a radiograph, these radiopaque structures are observed as white to light gray shades
- Less dense structures, such as periodontal spaces or sinuses, are said to be radiolucent
- These translucent areas allow much more penetration of the x-ray beam and appear as black or dark gray regions on the radiograph
- The two terms are relative

- Expected differences in shading on the radiograph along with anatomical landmarks are used as guidelines for mounting and interpretation of the radiograph and formation of a diagnosis

GENERAL RADIOGRAPHIC LANDMARKS

General anatomical landmarks related to teeth and surrounding tissues are used for mounting radiographs as are other specific maxillary and mandibular arch landmarks.

- On the crown of the tooth, the exterior hard enamel is radiopaque (white) and the underlying dentin is also to a lesser extent
- The pulp chamber is the radiolucent darker area in the middle of the tooth
- It is enveloped by dentin and radiolucent pulp or root canals run to the apex of the tooth
- The root is enclosed with a somewhat radiopaque substance called cementum
- The area surrounding the root, called the periodontal ligament space, should appear dark or radiolucent
- Bones in the area absorb x-rays and appear fairly radiopaque
- These bone landmarks include cancellous or relatively spongy bones (also known as the trabecular bone pattern), which are somewhat radiopaque and irregular looking
- They also include the denser and whiter-looking cortical bone or plate forming the tooth socket; there should be a radiopaque line representing the lamina dura or cortical bone around the tooth and periodontal ligament

MANDIBULAR ARCH LANDMARKS

There are many radiographic landmarks for the mandibular arch that can be utilized for mounting.

- These include various radiolucent foramens or natural openings, ridges, the mandibular canal, the retromolar area, and more
- Characteristic dark-appearing openings include the mental, lingual, and mandibular foramens at the roots of the premolar, the lingual side of the mandible at the midline, and the center of the ramus respectively
- The ramus is the dark relatively vertical area on each side of the lower jaw; at the top of it is the condyle and at the bottom is the coronoid process, both radiopaque
- The mandibular canal is a dark line running parallel to the apices of the molars
- A characteristic ridge is the internal or mylohyoid ridge which looks like a whitish area superimposed over the roots of the molars and premolars; there is also an external oblique ridge
- The chin area or symphysis forming the front of the mandible should be observed
- There should be a triangular section posterior to the molars called the retromolar area in which various tissue types are present

MAXILLARY ARCH LANDMARKS

There are many radiographic landmarks for the maxillary arch to use for mounting.

- The hard palate at the roof of the mouth is radiopaque; the radiolucent section at its midline is called the incisive foramen
- The nasal cavities or fossa are the dark areas above the tooth area in the front separated by the radiopaque nasal septum
- The maxillary sinuses are translucent areas on both sides above the apices of the teeth from about canine to molar areas

- There are several characteristic radiopaque areas near the maxillary molars
- Proceeding posteriorly, these include the zygomatic process, the tuberosity, and the hamulus
- The maxillary or median palatine suture should appear as a thin dark line between the central incisors
- The orbit or bone surrounding the eyeball may be seen
- An important part of the temporal bone, the depression on its lower border called the glenoid fossa, should be observed as well as the styloid process behind it, the mastoid process behind the ear, and the translucent external auditory meatus or auditory canal

ARTIFACTS ON RADIOGRAPHS

Artifacts or various conditions can be observed on radiographs.

- Any dense material such as orthodontic work, fillings for caries, implants or inserted pins, metallic restorations, bridges, or eyeglasses will appear as lighter or more radiopaque areas
- Deficits such as areas of developing caries or periodontal pockets will appear darker or more radiolucent than expected
- Supernumerary or extra teeth as well as unerupted or impacted teeth can be picked up by radiographs
- Pathological conditions can be diagnosed by looking at a radiograph
- Radiographic examination is useful even for the edentulous or toothless patient because it can pick up things like cysts, impacted teeth, or remaining root tips or bone fragments

EDENTULOUS RADIOGRAPHIC SURVEY

Radiographic surveys are taken on edentulous (toothless or partially toothless) individuals to identify artifacts, pathological conditions, and anatomical landmarks.

- Usually this is done to prepare for making dentures
- A full-mouth radiographic survey can often have a reduced number of films, for example, by omitting bite-wing radiographs
- Often occlusal or panoramic films are used
- Modifications are necessary to hold the films in place
- Cotton rolls are utilized to keep the film parallel to the alveolar ridge with the paralleling technique while leaving dentures in the other arch in place
- If the bisecting technique is used, the edge of the film is positioned a quarter inch inside the alveolar ridge crest
- Other modifications include greater vertical angulation and slightly decreased exposure time

ENDODONTIC-RELATED RADIOGRAPHS

Endodontics is the branch of dentistry dealing with pulp and periapical tissue diseases.

- Radiographs are generally taken during endodontic processes for reference
- The paralleling method is preferred to reduce distortion
- As there is a reamer tool placed in the root canal during these procedures, the individual keeps his or her mouth open, including during x-ray exposure
- The film must be positioned using a specialized device or hemostat

- The selected film, which is placed parallel on the tongue side of the tooth, should be large enough to cover the length of the tooth including the root apex
- The central x-ray beam is aimed perpendicular to the tooth

TEMPOROMANDIBULAR JOINT RADIOGRAPH

A specialized example of cephalometric radiography is the transcranial temporomandibular joint radiograph.

- Here the patient holds the large panoramic film cassette next to the side of his or her head, and the central x-ray is directed from above and behind the external auditory meatus or ear canal on the opposite side
- The purpose is to look at the primary structures comprising the temporomandibular joint area and their relationship
- The TMJ radiograph can be taken with a closed or open mouth
- The landmarks to look for are the condyle and glenoid fossa
- With the mouth closed, the condyle or posterior projection of the ramus of the mandible should be in close contact with the glenoid fossa, the depression on the lower border of the temporal bone of the maxilla
- The condyle should be cushioned by fibrous connective tissue called the meniscus or articular disc
- If the mouth is open in the picture, the condyle and meniscus should be further forward but still in close contact with the area further forward on the maxilla, the articular eminence

IMPRESSION TRAY TYPES

Impression trays are used to document tooth areas.

- They can be used for things such as diagnosing, making dental tools (e.g., a temporary dental crown), or developing an indirect casting
- Commercially-available stock or preformed trays are used for preliminary and final impressions and temporary needs
- They are sold in various sizes and materials including metal, Styrofoam and tough plastic
- Impression trays can cover the full arch, a half arch (quadrant tray), or just the front teeth (section tray)
- Some are perforated so that the impression material bonds with the tray
- Customized trays specially made for an individual are generally made of lightweight resins, either light-cured acrylic or thermoplastic
- They are used for final impressions, making temporary restorations, or vital bleaching (external surface teeth whitening)

PRELIMINARY IMPRESSIONS

An impression is a negative copy of teeth and adjacent structures.

- Preliminary impressions are utilized in the following ways: as diagnostic models; for preparation of orthodontic and dental appliances, for provisional dental crowns and the like; as records prior to and after treatment, and often as preparation for custom impressions
- Preliminary impressions created by the dentist or assistant (if legally allowed in that state) are usually made of alginate, a hydrocolloid comprised of potassium alginate and other compounds

- Alginate comes as a powder to which an equal amount of water must be added
- As water is added, the material first goes through a sol or solution phase that is liquid or semi-liquid, and then it proceeds to a gel or semisolid phase
- Typically, 2 or 3 scoops of powder and equal measures of water are used for mandibular or maxillary impressions
- Depending on whether the formulation is a normal set or fast set, the working time for making an impression is only 2 or 1¼ minutes respectively
- Additionally, normal and fast sets have setting times of only 4½ or 1 to 2 minutes respectively

ALGINATE IMPRESSION STEPS

As discussed elsewhere, alginate has short working and setting times.

- The dentist or assistant should be positioned so that insertion can be done quickly and with control after its preparation
- The impression tray containing the alginate mixture is turned a bit initially in order to place a corner of it into the patient's mouth
- The person's cheek should be moved out of the way while the tray is slid into the mouth and centered over the teeth
- The back part of the tray should be seated before the front part in order to the alginate from flowing into the mouth and throat
- The tray should be pushed into place very gently
- Then, the person's lips are pulled out around the tray which is held securely in place until the alginate sets

DIAGNOSTIC CASTS

A diagnostic cast is a positive mock-up of the teeth and surrounding structures created by filling in the impression with model plaster or dental stone.

- Model plaster is the weaker material and can be more easily trimmed off; it is related to plaster of Paris
- Dental stone is more robust and is the material of choice for preparation of things such as retainers or custom trays
- Both model plaster and dental stone contain gypsum, but a higher proportion of water is added to set model plaster than dental stone or its stronger relative high-strength stone
- Setting time is dependent on a number of factors, including the type of gypsum, the water-powder ratio, length and speed of mixing, water temperature, and humidity present
- Setting time is speeded up with a lower water-powder ratio, long or intense mixing, water temperature above about room temperature, or on a humid day
- Diagnostic casts are poured by the double-pour, box-and-pour, or inverted-pour methods
- They are trimmed and finished using an appliance called a model trimmer
- The end-product has two portions, an anatomic part showing the teeth, mucosa and muscle attachments (2/3) and an art portion or base (1/3)

FINAL IMPRESSIONS

Final impressions should provide more precise definition of the teeth and surrounding structures of interest than preliminary impressions.

- Occasionally alginate is used for final impressions, more often elastomeric impression materials are chosen
- Two compounds are mixed together to create the final elastomeric material, a base and a catalyst
- The various choices are defined by their viscosity or capacity to flow; light, regular, and heavy body materials are increasingly thick with the latter being the most commonly used
- There are 4 basic types of final impression materials available: polysulfide, polyether, condensation silicone, and addition silicone
- In terms of stiffness and stability, the best choice is addition stone, followed by polyether

PREPARATION AND TAKING IMPRESSION

Mixing time is a minute or less for all final impression materials.

- Setting time averages 6 minutes (or slightly more) for all except polysulfide which takes 10 to 20 minutes to set
- If the base and catalyst come as two pastes, they can be mixed either by swirling them together and smoothing them with a spatula or by using an automix system
- The automix system consists of extruder units with cartridges of the base and catalyst, which are mixed when a trigger is squeezed
- Usually the tooth for which the impression is being taken is segregated by a retraction system, rinsed and dried
- Then, a recently-mixed light-body impression material is inserted into the sulcus, around the tooth, and into adjacent areas
- The heavy-body material is then mixed, put into the impression tray, and loaded in place over the other material
- After setting, the impression is removed, examined, disinfected, and placed in a labeled precaution bag for transport to the laboratory
- Making final impressions is usually a two person job with the assistant doing the mixing and the dentist doing the actual impression

OCCLUSAL REGISTRATIONS

Occlusal or bite registrations are impressions that document the centric relationship between a patient's maxillary and mandibular arches.

- The centric relationship is the position of optimally stable connection between occlusal surfaces of the two arches when the mouth is closed
- Bite registrations are generally made either of wax or paste neither of which flows very easily
- If wax is used, it is heated for softening and placed directly onto the occlusal surfaces
- The patient bites down lightly into the wax until it cools, and then the registration is removed and stored
- Pastes set quickly, are odorless and tasteless, and conform easily to biting
- Pastes usually come in 2 parts that must be mixed or as cartridges
- Again, they can be spread right over the teeth or put in a gauze tray, and then the patient bites down for the impression

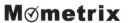

GINGIVAL RETRACTION

Gingival retraction uses a cord to briefly push the gingival tissue away from a tooth and broaden the sulcus.

- Gingival retraction cords are generally used to isolate a tooth to make a final impression
- The tooth should be dry and the quadrant should be separated off with cotton rolls
- A loop is made in the retraction cord, slid over the tooth, and then pushed into the sulcus in a clockwise motion with a special cord-packing device
- The end of the cord should end up on the facial side where it is either left sticking out or stuck into the sulcus
- After several minutes, the retraction cord is taken out, moving counterclockwise, with cotton pliers; the area is dried, new cotton rolls are applied, and the impression is procured quickly

OSHA BLOODBORNE/HAZARDOUS MATERIALS STANDARDS

The Occupational Safety and Health Administration (OSHA) originally published a comprehensive Bloodborne/Hazardous Materials Standard in 1991 that every dental employee must follow.

- The Standard covers all exposure issues related to blood and potentially infectious materials (OPIMs) such as saliva and other body fluids
- It details standard universal precautions for infection control, acceptable work practices, use of personal protective equipment, requirements for sharps containers and biohazardous waste disposal, engineering controls, housekeeping and laundry issues, hepatitis B vaccination, post exposure follow-up procedures, labeling and Safety Data Sheets (SDSs), training requirements and records, and employee responsibilities and recording of exposure
- Revisions to the Standard were added in 2001 that addressed issues such as employee input and use of a sharps injury log
- Compliance with the OSHA standard is mandatory with non-compliance fines up to $10,000 per employee

PPE

Personal protective equipment (PPE) is any type of protection used to prevent exposure to hazardous and infectious materials.

- Eye protection, gloves, and protective clothing are considered PPE and are required during possible exposure
- Eye protection is mandatory in instances where splashing of bodily fluids might occur
- Vinyl or latex gloves should be worn the hand might come in contact with infectious materials, and puncture resistant gloves are necessary when handling sharps
- Depending on the level of potential exposure, protective clothing can range from lab coats to fluid-resistant gowns to head, foot, and apron coverings that keep out fluids
- PPE should be kept on site, and protective clothing should also be laundered on site
- Contaminated clothing should be put in special red bags or tagged with biohazard labels
- Laundry employees in the facility should also use PPE and a sharps container

SHARPS CONTAINERS USE

Needles, other sharp instruments, and broken glass are all considered sharps.

- OSHA's Bloodborne/Hazardous Materials Standard requires that sharps containers be available in the work area
- These containers need to be puncture resistant, labeled or color coded, leak proof, and have closures
- Typically, these containers are made of hard red plastic with biohazard stickers and can be sealed and autoclaved when full
- Sharps should be put into these containers immediately after use
- Broken glass should be collected with a broom and dustpan first. In 2001 subsequent to the Needlestick Safety and Prevention Act and resultant revisions to the Standard, a sharps injury log for employees was mandated

ENGINEERING AND WORK PRACTICE CONTROLS

Sharps containers fall under the category of engineering and work practice controls, which also includes things such as splash guards on model trimmers, ventilation hoods for hazardous fumes, eye wash stations, needleless IVs, and self-sheathing needles

FLUIDS TYPES AND TISSUES

The OSHA Bloodborne/Hazardous Materials Standard covers blood and anything visibly contaminated with it as well as OPIMs, other potentially infectious materials.

- In dental practice, saliva is the most probable OPIM
- A variety of other fluids can be OPIMs, including cerebrospinal fluid, amniotic fluid, semen, vaginal secretions, synovial fluid surrounding joints, pericardial fluid from the heart, pleural fluid in the lung, or peritoneal fluid in the abdomen
- Tissues other than intact skin can be OPIMs. Cell, tissue and organ cultures, or solutions that contain human immunodeficiency virus (HIV) or hepatitis B virus (HBV) as well as similar products from experimental animals are considered OPIMs
- These viruses are two of the greatest exposure concerns
- For that reason, the Standard also mandates that free hepatitis B vaccination be made available to employees within 10 days and later if exposed
- HBV vaccination is a good general practice for any healthcare employee

EXPOSURE TO BLOODBORNE PATHOGENS PROCEDURES

An exposure incident report should be made with copies for the employee's confidential medical records and the healthcare professional (HCP) evaluating the worker.

- The report should include exposure route, the patient involved, and other relevant circumstances
- In offices with at least 11 employees, completion of OSHA forms 200 and 101 is also required
- The HBV and HIV status of both worker and patient should be obtained or if known communicated to the HCP
- Patient consent must be obtained for testing, which should be promptly performed unless declined
- Employee consent is also required before testing, which may be withheld or delayed up to 90 days

- The HCP coordinates this testing, gives the affected worker the results, provides counseling and prophylactic measures if indicated based on these results, and evaluates any medical problems that might develop
- Prophylaxis can include HBV vaccination if not done previously or chemoprophylaxis if HIV transmission is likely
- The HCP sends a written opinion to the employer who in turn must convey that to the employee within 15 days of evaluation

OSHA HAZARD COMMUNICATION STANDARD

The OSHA Hazard Communication Standard addresses use of hazardous chemicals.

- It mandates that new employees receive this type of safety training within 30 days of employment or before they are exposed to any of these chemicals as well as annually subsequently
- Safety training should include content in the Hazardous Communication Standard, spill cleanup procedures, reading of chemical labels, use of safety data sheets, chemical storage and inventory guidelines, disposal procedures for hazardous waste, and training certification documentation
- General OSHA laws and many elements that pertain to exposure to bloodborne pathogens should also be covered

CHEMICAL INVENTORY FORM

A chemical inventory form should be kept summarizing all hazardous chemicals used in the dental office.

- The form should have information about the hazard classification in terms of the relative health hazard presented, the degree of fire hazard possible, the reactivity, and the protective gear that should be used when handling each chemical
- For example, a zero usually represents a minimal health hazard, inability to burn, or a stable reactivity
- Slight, moderate, serious, or extreme hazards in each category might be labeled from 1 to 4
- Protective gear needed could be any combination of goggles, gloves, clothing, mask, and/or face shield
- The chemical inventory should also include information about the quantity in storage, the chemical's physical state, manufacturer's contacts, and other comments
- Physical state refers to whether the chemical is a liquid, solid or gas

CHEMICAL WARNING LABELS

Chemical warning labels use the National Fire Protection Association's color and number method and contain the same information needed on a chemical inventory form.

- A chemical warning label is diamond-shaped and has four quadrants of different colors
- Three quadrants have numbers indicating hazard level. The top quadrant is red indicating potential fire hazard (0 = non-combustible, 1 = combustible if heated, 2 = combustible liquid, 3 = flammable liquid, and 4 = flammable gas or extremely flammable liquid)
- The left triangle gives the potential health hazard (0 = no unusual hazard, 1 = possible irritant, 2 = harmful if inhaled, 3 = corrosive or toxic, and 4 = dangerous and possibly fatal)

- The right triangle indicates reactivity (0 = stable in water, 1 = possible reactivity if heated or mixed with water, 2 = unstable or possibly reactive if mixed with water, 3 = dangerous and possibly explosive with a spark or heating under confinement, and 4 = dangerous and explosive at room temperature)
- The bottom quadrant is white and will contain a letter if personal protective equipment is required

SAFETY DATA SHEETS

Safety data sheets or SDSs are manufacturer-provided sheets containing pertinent information about chemicals purchased.

- SDSs should be kept in a safety data manual or the information should be on the computer
- A SDS contains product and manufacturer identification, hazardous ingredients, physical data, fire and explosion potential, reactivity data, health hazard data, emergency and first aid procedures if in contact, spill or leak and waste disposal procedures, personal protection equipment needed, and any special precautions
- Physical data includes details like the solubility in water, vapor pressure and freezing and boiling points of the mixture
- Fire, reactivity, and health hazard information is generally more specific than that indicated on a chemical warning label
- Special precautions may address storage issues

Radiation Health and Safety

Techniques and Processes

TYPICAL INTRAORAL FILM

Intraoral films usually come in one of 5 sizes: No. 0 for children; a narrow No. 1 for front teeth; the adult size No. 2: No. 3 used for long bite-wing films; and occlusal or No. 4 films.

- A typical intraoral dental film packet consists of a sealed external plastic wrapper to eliminate moisture with black paper inside enclosing the dental film
- There is also a lead foil backing on the film that soaks up any excess radiation or scatter
- The lead foil backing is important because it thwarts film fogging
- It should always be positioned away from the x-ray beam during exposure
- The packet should indicate which side should be placed toward the tube
- Unexposed film should be kept at about 50 to 70 degrees Fahrenheit; refrigerator storage is acceptable
- After exposure and processing, the films are mounted and put in protective envelopes

RADIOGRAPHIC ANGULATION IMPACT

Incorrect vertical angulation can result in elongation or foreshortening errors.

- Both of these are more likely to occur with the bisecting technique
- Elongation is the radiographic appearance of overly lengthened teeth due to too little vertical angulation
- Foreshortening is the opposite
- Teeth appear short due to too much vertical angulation
- Erroneous horizontal angulation can result in overlapping
- Overlapping occurs because the central x-ray was not directed at the interproximal areas and/or the angle between film and beam is not exactly 90 degrees
- Image distortion can result from things like bent or curved films
- If the ray is not directly centered over the film, an error called cone cutting can transpire
- Incorrect machine settings can result in underexposed or overexposed film
- Patient or equipment movement during exposure can result in blurred images
- Clear films indicate lack of radiation exposure
- Other common errors are double exposures on the same film, radiopaque areas due to metals like eyeglasses, or a herringbone pattern due to backward film placement

FILM PROCESSING ERRORS

Light film images usually result from film processing errors such as shortened developing time, a developer temperature that is too low, depleted developing solution, or fixation errors

- Images that are overly dark are usually due to overdevelopment or high developer temperature
- Fogged films (which appear gray and do not show much detail or contrast) are due to such things as improper storage or light leaks during processing

Copyright © Mometrix Media. You have been licensed one copy of this document for personal use only. Any other reproduction or redistribution is strictly prohibited. All rights reserved.
This content is provided for test preparation purposes only and does not imply an endorsement by Mometrix of any particular political, scientific, or religious point of view.

- Processing errors can produce partial images (through lack of contact with adequate solution), frayed or scratched films, streaks (usually caused by automatic processing rollers), or white spots (due to trapped air bubbles)
- There are a number of film artifacts that can occur as a result of processing errors, such as brownish stains from inadequate rinsing, white or black spots from unresolved fixer or developer, or fingerprint smudges
- Films that have been sequentially exposed to high and then low temperatures can undergo a phenomenon called reticulation where the emulsion swells and then shrivels; the resultant films appear dry and cracked

MANUAL PROCESSING ROOM

The manual processing room or darkroom for radiographic processing must be set up such that all sources of light leaks are excluded during processing.

- There should be a safelight installed above the manual processing tank and areas where films are unwrapped, mounted or viewed
- Radiographic films are sensitive to the longer wavelengths in the blue-green spectrum
- Therefore, the safelight should have filters either in the red-orange or orange spectrum for intraoral films or red spectrum for extraoral films where intensifying screens have been used
- A good overall choice is the Kodak GBX-2 safelight filter
- The room should be a light color
- The switch for turning on the overhead lighting during non-processing or reading times should be away from the area
- The manual processing room typically contains a stainless steel tank with two inserts for developer and fixer (left and right respectively) within a water bath
- There are associated gauges and controls, a silver recovery unit, storage units for equipment such as solution stirring rods, film dryer, processing racks to hang films, a view box for observation, cleaning supplies, and an accurate timer

PREPARATION AND TEMPERATURE CONSTRAINTS

A manual processing tank usually has inserts for developer on the left and fixer on the right.

- These solutions are generally provided as liquid concentrates which are added to each tank and then diluted with water to an indicator line on the tank
- Water is also circulated through the water bath
- Ideally the temperature of each component should be between 68°F to 70°F
- At those temperatures, optimal developer times are 4½ and 4 minutes respectively
- Higher temperatures mandate shorter and conversely lower temperatures require longer developer times
- Chemicals in the solutions may be unstable if the temperature is above 80°F or below 60°F
- Solutions should be replaced at least every 3 weeks to a month
- If they get low, a 50:50 mix of developer/water can be added to that tank; additional fixer should be added undiluted
- Test films should also be run when solutions are changed and again daily for comparison

PROCESSING SOLUTIONS CHEMICAL COMPOSITION AND DISPOSAL

Developer solution is designed to decrease the exposed area of the emulsion on a film.

- It has an alkaline pH above 7
- Developer consists of the reducing agents hydroquinone and elon, the alkaline vehicle sodium carbonate, the preservative sodium sulfite, a slowing agent called potassium bromide, and distilled water
- The reducing agents are the essential ingredients as they blacken the silver halide crystals to create film contrast
- Fixer solution is used to terminate the developing process and get rid of free crystals
- Fixer consists of sodium hyposulfite (thiosulfite) (which strips off the crystals), acetic acid (which terminates the development), the preservative sodium sulfite, potassium alum (for hardening and shrinking of the gelatin), and water
- In both cases, sodium sulfite acts as a preservative by preventing oxidation
- Used solutions should be disposed of by placing them in containers and having them removed by a biohazardous waste company according to OSHA standards
- This is imperative for the used fixer solution, which contains silver
- Film packets must also be put aside in containers for metal recycling as they contain lead

RADIOGRAPHS UTILIZING A MANUAL TANK

Exposed radiographs are handled with clean, dry hands (or gloves if contaminated).

- The processing zone should be clean
- The solutions should be checked for temperature with a thermometer and for volume to determine if they need topping off
- Dedicated stirring rods should be used to mix each in the morning and again in the afternoon
- The x-ray rack is labeled
- At this point, white lights are turned off and safelights on before films are taken out of their wrappers and attached to the racks
- The film rack is put in the developer tank and moved around to get rid of bubbles
- The top of the tank is attached and the timer is set for development (4½ minutes if the temperature is the ideal 68°F)
- The rack is taken out at the chosen time with excess dripping back into the solution
- The rack is rinsed in the circulating water area between the two solutions for 30 seconds
- The film rack is then put in the fixing solution for 10 minutes; films can be viewed briefly before complete fixation after 3 minutes
- After fixing, the radiographs are rinsed as before but for 20 minutes
- This is followed by drying with an electric film dryer for 15 to 20 minutes and mounting

AUTOMATIC RADIOGRAPH PROCESSORS

Automatic processors use a succession of rollers to transfer the film through developer, fixer, water, and drying compartments before dropping the processed film onto a tray.

- Automatic processing takes less time than manual because the temperature is much higher, somewhere between 82°F and 95°F
- Most automatic processors have another advantage, daylight loading units, eliminating the need for a safelighting setup

- The processing solutions used are slightly different as they contain chemicals that inhibit emulsion sticking to the rollers (making them incompatible with manual processing)
- The main drawback with automatic processing is that maintenance of the units is crucial
- If an automatic processor is used, it needs to be warmed up and ready before use
- Exposed radiographs and two cups are placed into the daylight loader with clean, dry hands
- After gloving, the technician takes out each radiograph within the holder separating exposed films and empty packets into different cups
- He or she then removes the gloves and slowly delivers each film individually or on a holder into the processor and collects and mounts them afterwards

RADIOGRAPHS DUPLICATION

Original radiographs should be retained at the dental office in case it is necessary to duplicate radiographs for legal and other purposes.

- The dental assistant makes duplicates using special duplicating film and a duplicating machine
- The duplicating film produces direct positive images and has emulsion only one side
- Duplicating machines are relatively small devices with internal light sources
- An original radiograph is positioned on the duplicator with the dot upward
- Using safelight environment, the duplicating film is then placed on top of the radiograph touching it with the emulsion side down
- The lid is closed and fastened
- Then, the machine is turned on and a very short 4 to 5 second timed exposure is taken
- The duplicating film is taken out under safelight and processed either automatically or manually

MOUNTING RADIOGRAPHS TECHNIQUES

The American Dental Association endorses labial mounting of radiographs.

- This means that the mount is done with the raised dot or convex side upward similar to the way the radiograph is taken, creating a view into the mouth with the person's right side on the left side of the mount and vice versa
- Lingual mounting places the concave side or depression upwards giving the impression of looking outward from the oral cavity
- In either case, mounts should be firm enough (usually plastic or cardboard) to hold the films and have the desired number of windows
- Mounts should always be labeled with the person's name and exposure date
- Mounting is usually done utilizing a view box
- Radiographs are assembled with all dots either up or down and then sorted by type
- For a typical window assortment of 4 bite-wings, 6 anterior, and 8 posterior films, the bite-wing radiographs are usually mounted first followed by the anterior and then the posterior
- The goal is to make sure that the smile pattern or curve of Spee is evident for both jaws
- Characteristics of types of teeth, discussed elsewhere, are used for identification

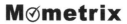

COIN AND STEP WEDGE TESTS

These tests are forms of quality assurance.

- The "coin test" is a method of monitoring the darkroom for light leaks. The test should be performed every month. In the film processing zone, a penny or other coin is left on top of an unexposed, unwrapped radiographic film under safelight conditions for 2 to 3 minutes and then processed as usual. If the silhouette of the coin is visible on the film after processing, then either there is a white light leak into the room or the safelight is not satisfactory
- The "step wedge test" uses either commercially-available or homemade lead step wedges. The latter can be made from the lead foil of x-ray film packets. This test is used to evaluate processing solution over time by comparing the density or darkness of daily test films. Usually 20 radiographs are exposed when solutions are changed. Then, every day one of the radiographs is processed and compared to the initial one in terms of density shown in the middle of the films.

DENTAL RADIOGRAPHY EQUIPMENT QA

The American Academy of Dental Radiology has published a number of recommendations for quality assurance (QA) related to dental radiography equipment.

- Various parameters are usually monitored yearly by state agencies
- Every month the x-ray machine's timer should be checked for accuracy using a spin top
- An exposure is taken with the spin top spinning on top of a film
- This produces an image with a number of dots that should equal the number of impulses chosen on the x-ray machine
- Another recommended monthly test is a check for milliamperage, which uses the step wedge to compare shades of light, medium, and dark areas; a variance in shading of more than two steps from previous exposures indicates the need for mA adjustment
- The kilovoltage output should also be checked by aiming the PID at the dosimeter and exposing it; the dosimeter reading should match the indicated kV output
- Other parameters, some of which need to be checked yearly by the state, include the half value layer (HVL), focal spot size, beam placement and size, radiation output, reproducibility, and tubehead stability

ADVANCED IMAGING SYSTEMS

Digital imaging or computed dental radiography is rapidly becoming the standard in many dental practices.

- The exposures are taken in a standard manner with x-ray machinery, but the images are processed with special equipment connected to a computer for digitization and rapid viewing, printing, storing, augmentation, and even transmission to others
- There are specialized image plates with sensors used for the exposure
- Afterwards, the plate is mounted on a carousel, scanned in a scanner, and sent to the computer
- A system such as the DenOptix Imaging Cycle can produce computer images of as many as 8 plates in less than 2 minutes
- Digital equipment is expensive and a learning curve is involved, but there are many advantages in terms of enhancement, storage, and maintenance

- Another technique that might be used is computed tomography or CT scanning, which also uses ionizing radiation but generates a multidimensional image on a computer monitor
- Magnetic resonance imaging or MRI, which utilizes low energy electromagnetic radiation, is primarily employed to diagnose temporomandibular joint disease

RADIOGRAPH QUALITY FACTORS

Radiographic quality is influenced by four factors.

- The first is contrast or the range of lightness and darkness displaced. Good contrast in a radiograph differentiates between the whiteness in radiopaque areas such restorations, blackness in radiolucent or unoccupied areas, and various shades of gray for other objects. Contrast is dependent on the kVp or kilovoltage peak; kVp is inversely related to degree of contrast
- The next factor is density or the general darkness of the radiograph. Density is directly related to the amount of radiation in contact with the film and is primarily controlled by the mA or milliamperage supplied. Density is also directly related to kVp and exposure time
- Patient body size or thickness can affect density inversely. Processing times and temperatures affect density too. Good radiographs have good image detail which is related to contrast and density
- Quality radiographs have little image distortion

IMAGE DISTORTION FACTORS

Image distortion has three main sources: incorrect object-film distance, improper source-film distance, or movement.

- The object-film distance (OFD) is the space between the object being photographed and the film
- Image distortion, primarily a lack of clarity, can occur when the radiographic film is put too far away from the teeth during exposure
- The source-film distance is the gap between the x-ray source and the film
- This parameter is related to the length of the position indicator device
- Longer PIDs and close placement of the film to the end of the PID produce less image distortion
- Position indicator devices or PIDs come in various lengths, typically either 8, 12, or 16 inches
- Longer PIDs generate less spread or divergence of the x-ray beam, resulting in less magnification of the image
- Thus, the longer 16-inch size is usually preferred
- The other factor that can produce image distortion or lack of sharpness is any type of movement by the patient, the tubehead, or the film

X-ray Physics and Safety

X-RAYS

X-rays are a form of radiation or electromagnetic energy.

- All forms of electromagnetic energy travel in waves and have characteristic wavelengths
- Wavelength is inversely is related to the wave frequency and energy
- The energy forms utilized in dental radiography, x-rays and gamma rays, have shorter wavelengths, higher frequencies, and higher energy than other forms such as ultraviolet radiation from the sun, infrared energy, or electricity
- All electromagnetic energy forms proceed in a straight line at the speed of light, 186,000 miles/second. X-ray photons (discrete quantities of energy) proceed in a straight line but can be redirected through interaction with matter

RADIATION TYPES

An x-ray machine directs the central beam of x-rays from the tubehead toward the area being documented; this is the primary radiation.

- There can also be unwanted leakage radiation dispersing from other areas of the tubehead
- There are two types of radiation that result from interaction with matter and have different paths
- There is deflected secondary radiation that occurs when the primary radiation x-ray photons strike atoms in matter and cause ionization
- Some orbital electrons in the matter are lost and others become positively charged
- Scatter radiation, referring to that averted from its path during interaction with matter, can result

POSSIBLE BIOLOGICAL EFFECTS

Radiation, including x-rays, can have permanent and sometimes hereditary biological effects.

- If a person is exposed to radiation in areas that contain reproductive cells, permanent genetic changes can occur through generation of mutations or changes in the DNA (deoxyribonucleic acid)
- Most other interactions between radiation and matter result in somatic changes
- While somatic changes are not transmitted to progeny, they can present genuine health problems
- Certain tissue types are more sensitive to the effects of radiation than others
- In particular, these radiosensitive cells are those that are rapidly dividing and/or non-specific such as lymphoid or bone marrow cells
- Oral radiographs can present exposure to moderately sensitive areas (e.g., the skin and oral mucosa), somewhat sensitive areas (e.g., connective tissue and developing bones), and less sensitive areas (e.g. salivary glands, mature bone, and thyroid)
- The least sensitive tissue types are those that are not actively undergoing much cell division such as the muscles and nerves
- Effects of all types of radiation are cumulative and often latent in appearance

RADIATION MEASUREMENT AND GUIDELINES FOR EXPOSURE

Radiation is measured in terms of the quantity of ionizing radiation absorbed or the amount of exposure.

- Both are related to the unit originally defined, the roentgen or R, the amount of radiation ionizing one cubic centimeter of air
- The radiation absorbed dose (rad) can also be expressed in Gray (GY) units, with 100 rads = 1 GY
- Rads are related to the exposure dose or dose equivalent defined as either the roentgen equivalent man (rem) or sievert (Sv). 100 rems = 1 Sv
- Various forms of energy and affected tissues are given a unit of relative biological effectiveness (rbe), which for diagnostic dental practice is 1 rbe for x-rays
- Dental and office personnel and patients are required to receive as low as reasonably achievable (ALARA) amounts of radiation
- This translates to a maximum permissible dose (MPD) by broadest definitions for occupational exposure for dental personnel of 0.05 Sv or 5 rems yearly or 100 rems weekly
- Pregnant employees and other personnel should receive only a tenth of that amount, and the International Commission on Radiological Protection suggests a lower limit of 2 rems yearly

DENTAL X-RAY UNIT

The dental x-ray unit consists of a control panel, an arm assembly, and a tubehead.

- The control panel typically has either digital or manual settings for the milliamperage, kilovoltage and time
- Milliamperage (mA) refers to a unit of measurement of electrical current, which is directly related to the amount of radiation delivered
- The milliamperage control usually also serves as an on/off switch
- Typical settings used range from 10 to 15 mA
- Kilovoltage (kV) is a measurement of potential difference or degree of penetration
- The kilovoltage is inversely related to exposure time needed and also affects the radiographic quality
- Typical settings range from 70 to 90 kV
- Switches operating the timer are usually external to the unit to limit operator exposure
- The amount of radiation exposure to the patient is expressed in milliamperage seconds (mAs), calculated as mA delivered times number of seconds

ARM ASSEMBLY AND TUBEHEAD

An x-ray unit has an arm assembly that is affixed to the wall with a flexible section used to place the tubehead.

- The tubehead is connected to the flexible extension and is the source of the x-rays
- There are two transformers offering different voltages as well as the actual x-ray tube in the tubehead
- There is a vacuum in the x-ray tube to eliminate interactions with other molecules
- Negatively-charged electrons are generated at the cathode (-) end of the leaded glass x-ray tube using a focusing cup of molybdenum with a tungsten filament

- This focuses the flow of electrons to the other end, the anode (+), containing a tungsten target with a focal spot which redirects the resulting x-ray stream out through a non-leaded window or aperture
- Excess heat is removed through a copper stem into oil in the tubehead
- There is a metal filter there that sorts out certain x-rays
- The desired rays for the central beam are those that have short wavelengths (hard x-rays)
- Further filtration is done by a lead disc with an opening called a collimator
- The x-ray beam exits through the PID or position indicator device (also known as the cone)

RADIOGRAPHY RESPONSIBILITIES

The manufacturer of the x-ray unit has federally-mandated responsibilities.

- These include clear controls, a separate control switch, and use of lead in the lining of the PID and on the collimator
- Further regulations insist on a maximum useful beam diameter of 2.75 inches upon exit from the collimator and filtration through at least 2.5 mm of aluminum if the kilovoltage is greater than 70
- The dentist's responsibilities include safe office design, conscientious use of x-ray prescription, supervision of machine maintenance and repair, and employment and supervision of adequately trained and certified assistants
- The dental assistant, who usually takes the actual radiographs, is in charge of preparing the patient through use of a lead apron with thyroid collar and also labeling and storing the radiographs properly
- Dental assistants are required to be educated in exposure and developing principles and techniques, aseptic procedures, radiation safety, and quality assurance
- The patient also has some responsibilities such as providing up-to-date information about his or her health and radiation history

RADIATION EXPOSURE REDUCTION

The choice of film, shape of position indicator device, choice of filters, and lead apron use can all affect radiation exposure.

- Films are usually classified according to speed as D, E, or F
- The fastest F-speed film (such as Kodak InSight) can decrease radiation exposure 20% relative to an E-speed film like Ektaspeed and even more relative to a D-speed type
- PIDs that are rectangular in shape eliminate much more radiation than those with round collimators
- Tissue exposure to radiation can be reduced by about half with use of proper filters, in particular rare earth filters
- Use of a lead apron by the patient virtually cuts out all exposure to reproductive areas, and thyroid exposure is cut in half with the addition of a thyroid collar
- All dental assistants who take radiographs must wear dosimeter or film badges that check radiation exposure

DENTAL X-RAY FILM COMPOSITION

Dental x-ray films have several layers.

- In the center there is transparent base made of cellulose acetate about 0.2 mm thick
- The base, which has a blue tint to improve image quality, is merely a support structure for the emulsion attached by an adhesive to either side of the base
- Emulsion consists of silver halide (usually bromide) crystals embedded in gelatin
- The silver halide crystals retain the energy from exposure in a so-called latent image, which is only revealed through development
- Basically, during development, added chemicals react with the exposed regions appearing black or radiolucent while unexposed areas wash off and are lighter
- There is also an outer protective coating on either side of a dental x-ray film

Orthodontic Procedures

Techniques

OFFICE SETUP

An orthodontic office should be setup with separate areas or rooms for the business office, the reception area, staff rooms, record-keeping areas, the darkroom, a laboratory, the orthodontist's private office, and a treatment area.

- The treatment area is usually designed as an open alcove with a number of dental chairs and units
- The head of the orthodontic team is the orthodontist, a dentist who has finished an additional two years of schooling in the field of orthodontics or jaw and teeth irregularities and malalignments
- The orthodontist is in charge of patient examination, diagnosis, and orthodontic treatment
- There are usually a number of office staff members, including a receptionist to greet patients, an office coordinator to ensure a smooth office operation, and possibly other business personnel to take care of financial or other aspects
- There may be one or more laboratory technicians who pour and trim diagnostic models and casts and create custom appliances and retainers
- Lastly, there is at least one orthodontic assistant working with the dentist in a variety of capacities

COA

A Certified Orthodontic Assistant (COA) is an individual who has passed a specialized examination given by DANB, the Dental Assisting National Board. Some state Boards of Dentistry also give credentialing examinations.

- An orthodontic assistant's duties related to direct patient contact include greeting and dismissing the individual, general chairside assisting and teeth cleaning at certain treatment points, co-presentation with the dentist of the treatment plan, and instructing the patient on oral hygiene and appliance wear and care
- Responsibilities for activities directly related to treatment if allowed by state Dental Practice Act include prefitting of bands prior to cementation, removing surplus cement from bands and brackets, application of sealants for bonding, checking appliances, situating and removing arch wires and ligatures, and band and bracket removal
- The assistant's responsibilities related to diagnosis include taking and processing of any needed intraoral and extraoral radiographs, performing the tracing on cephalometric ones, and generating study model impressions
- He or she is also accountable for inventory and supply maintenance

ORTHODONTIC TREATMENTS

Orthodontic treatment can be done to preserve or create functional occlusion, for facial esthetics, to remove problems that may disturb normal tooth or facial structure growth, or to correct existing defects in the oral-facial area.

- Much is considered preventive and interceptive, meaning that it is done to prevent later malocclusion
- Actions falling into this category include early correction of bad habits, identification of deviations, and observation of growth patterns of teeth and bones
- Preventive orthodontics also includes extraction of teeth to prevent overcrowding, taking out primary teeth to make room for permanent ones, doing restorations for tooth loss prevention, and putting in space maintainers if teeth are temporarily missing
- These activities are often performed in conjunction with or by a general dentist
- The other category, corrective orthodontics, involves correction of existing oral and facial deformities
- The techniques of corrective orthodontics are fixed appliance attachment to teeth, creation of removable appliances, or in severe instances orthognathic surgery
- Most corrective measures are done on children during the last stage of mixed dentition

ORTHODONTIC APPLIANCES

Orthodontic appliances have two functions, movement of teeth by application of force and keeping teeth in position.

- Tooth movement is dependent on the magnitude, time of application, direction, and distribution of the force
- Appliance use creates tooth movement via resorption, the removal of unnecessary tissues, and it maintains teeth positioning through creation of new cells or deposition
- When an orthodontic appliance applies pressure to the periodontal ligament, the blood supply is somewhat reduced on one side, triggering breakdown of surrounding bone cells called osteoclasts
- On the other side, ligaments become elongated and taut, creating space for other bone cells called osteoblasts to insert new bone (osteogenesis) to maintain positioning. This process can take up to a year

PATIENT'S INITIAL VISIT

The initial or preorthodontic patient visit is primarily diagnostic in nature.

- An inclusive medical and dental history should be taken
- The dentist should do a comprehensive clinical examination of the patient concentrating on the face, jaws and teeth; in particular, he or she should look for degree of symmetry, teeth and jaw characteristics and relationships, the angle classification of occlusion, and abnormalities in the oral cavity
- Panoramic radiographs are indicated for a global view of dentition and other areas such as the temporomandibular joint as well as cephalometric radiographs because their side view gives information about the jaw, teeth, and growth patterns
- Cephalometric exposures should be done periodically later; tracings are done on them manually or by computer to look at growth patterns or areas needing work
- Photographs (including full frontal and profile views of the face as well as intraoral pictures from various angles) should be taken before and after orthodontic work

- These are done to look at symmetry and balance
- Finally, diagnostic study models or casts should be taken; an alginate impression is taken, trimmed, finished and kept as for reference

CONSULTATION APPOINTMENT

Subsequent to the patient's initial diagnostic appointment, a consultation appointment is arranged with the individual. Patients 17 years of age or younger are required to have a parent present.

- During the consultation, the orthodontist presents a diagnosis and treatment plan including time and procedures involved and probable costs to the patient
- All pertinent diagnostic tests or models should be available for perusal
- Depending on the patient's age, treatment plans may have more than one phase
- For example, children without full permanent teeth may need removable appliances before they get fixcd ones
- If the patient is amenable to the treatment plan, he or she (or the parents) sign a consent form and formulate payment plans at this time

ORTHODONTIC BANDS, BRACKETS, AND ARCH WIRES

Orthodontic bands, brackets, and arch wires are the primary components of fixed orthodontic appliances or braces.

- Orthodontic bands are fine bands made of stainless steel that are cemented to posterior teeth
- Other attachments like brackets are generally set onto bands
- Brackets are utilized on both back and front teeth to grasp and transfer force from the arch wire to facilitate tooth movement
- They are soldered onto the bands or bonded to the teeth
- Brackets are made from either stainless steel or if they are placed on anterior teeth possibly ceramic or acrylic materials
- Arch wires are thin wires that are installed starting at the back molars through brackets for application of force
- As treatment proceeds and teeth move, arch wire positioning is generally modified

LIGATURE WIRES, PLASTIC RINGS, BUCCAL TUBES, SPRINGS, AND ELASTICS PURPOSES

These are all devices used in conjunction with bands, brackets, and arch wires for fixed appliances.

- Extremely thin ligature wires or plastic rings (elastic ties) are employed to keep the arch wire in the bracket by wrapping around the latter
- A common variation is the elastic chain, which can be used on several adjoining teeth
- There are also newly developed ligature ties that can deliver fluoride to the teeth and reduce calcium loss
- Buccal tubes, cylindrical metal attachments, are generally soldered to bands on the outer surface of molars; they are used for arch wire attachment
- Springs may be connected to the main arch wire to either provide additional pressure to specific teeth (finger spring) or affect specific spaces (coil spring)
- There are numerous types of elastic bands and threads that are used to generate additional force for tooth movement
- These elastics are clipped onto the band or brackets

SPECIAL FIXED APPLIANCES

Lingual, or invisible, braces are affixed to the lingual instead of the outer side of the teeth.

- While they may be more esthetically pleasing, they are tricky to install and maintain
- Lingual arch wires are generally used for children to preserve the arch by keeping teeth in place until permanent teeth erupt; they are installed lingually instead of being placed on the outer surface
- Space maintainers are appliances consisting of a band welded to a wire ring; they are used in children who have lost a deciduous tooth to preserve a place for the permanent tooth to come in correctly
- Another type of fixed device is a palatal separating appliance, which is used to broaden the mid-palatal suture
- These appliances are made of acrylic pieces cemented to back teeth on each side of the arch separated by an adjustable screw in the middle
- They are generally used for about 2 to 3 weeks until bone tissue develops

REMOVABLE APPLIANCES

Headgear is designed to be worn for a certain number of hours daily and usually consists of some type of strap and facebow that is fastened to buccal tubes.

- Headgear is employed for a variety of reasons, including application of force for tooth movement, control of cranial-facial bone development, or as an adjunct to fixed appliances
- Retainers are specially-made acrylic and/or metal devices used after removal of fixed appliances to keep teeth in place
- Tooth positioners have similar roles but are made of flexible rubber or supple plastic fitting over the crowns
- There are also a number of functional appliances utilized before insertion of fixed ones
- Some of the most common functional appliances are activators; examples include the Bionator, Herbst and Frankel appliances
- These are used for various purposes, including direction of tooth movement, changing the growth rate or width of an arch, modification of cranial-facial skeletal growth, or reduction of overbite
- Invisalign Aligners are also removable appliances

INVISALIGN ALIGNERS

Invisalign Aligners are a series of thin, clear, relatively rigid custom-made removable orthodontic appliances that fit over the patient's teeth.

- Each Aligner is worn at least 2 weeks and eventually replaced with another one as tooth movement occurs
- Aligners are designed to be worn at least 22 hours a day and taken out only for meals and tooth brushing and flossing
- The manufacturer Align Technology offers certification programs on their use
- Inclusive records including full-mouth or panoramic radiographs, PVS impressions of both arches, a PVS bite, and intra- and extraoral photographs are sent with a diagnosis and prescription to Align which fashions a three-dimensional model of the person's teeth and ClinCheck software
- The latter is a virtual depiction of the patient's teeth prior to and throughout the process of potential Aligner use

- The dentist assesses the ClinCheck file, makes changes if desired, and approves the plan
- After approval, Align makes a set of resin models for all of the Aligners, creates customized proprietary Aligners from them, and sends them to the dentist
- After trying the first set for two weeks, the patient is usually given several sets to change at approximately 2 week intervals

ORTHODONTIC WORK PLIERS

There are numerous pliers and other types of instruments used in orthodontic work.

- All pliers have similar outward-curving handles but different heads
- The Coons ligature tying pliers are both used to maneuver ligature wire
- The posterior band removing pliers and band contouring pliers are both utilized primarily on posterior bands, for removal or shaping respectively
- Band removing pliers have a padded end that is placed on the buccal cusp and a blade that is used to pull up against the gum side of the band to unseat it
- Arch wires are positioned with the Weingart utility pliers, which have matching curving aspects at the gripping points
- Arch wire ends are usually cut off with a distal-end cutting pliers, which have thick bent ends with cutting-edges
- Three-prong pliers are employed to adjust and bend wire and clasps
- Springs and other loops are made from wire utilizing either tweed-loop pliers or bird beak pliers, which have short triangular ends
- The adhesive-removing pliers have a sharp lip that should be used on the gingival side of the bracket and a nylon tip directed to the occlusal edge of the bracket

ORTHODONTIC INSTRUMENTS

Several instruments are used to maneuver ligature wire.

- The Mathieu needle holder is used to tie the wire and secure elastic ligatures
- A ligature director, which is straight in appearance, is utilized to push the twisted ligature wire ends into the interproximal spaces; it usually has one straight and one curved pronged edge
- There are also pin and ligature or light wire cutters that are used to cut the wire
- The molar bands are seated with either a band seater or a bite stick band seater (or band biter)
- The latter has a flat end and employs the force of occlusion for seating
- A band driver or pusher with a small, flattened disc head on one end is used for further positioning
- There are also a variety of available bracket placement tweezers or forceps that are employed to hold brackets while they are being put into place

SEPARATORS PURPOSE

Separators are used to prepare teeth for application of orthodontic bands.

- They are only worn a few days
- They can be made of elastic, steel springs, or brass wire, and are temporarily put between contact surfaces of teeth to widen the gap for later bands
- Some states allow the dental assistant to apply and remove elastic separators

- The elastic separators can be placed with either separating pliers or dental floss using gloves and aseptic technique
- A mouth mirror is used to observe the mouth
- If separating pliers are utilized, each elastic band is compressed tightly in the pliers
- The pliers are then shoved between the teeth using a forward and backward motion and one side of the band is introduced into the interproximal space
- The dental floss method uses two lengths of floss through the separator to stretch and position the separator; after placement, the dental floss is pulled out
- Elastic separators are removed before actual band placement by using one end of a scaler or explorer while bracing with a finger lightly pulling toward the occlusal surface for release

STEEL SPRING SEPARATORS OR BRASS WIRE

A steel spring separator typically has short and long legs with a coiled area in between.

- The long leg has a curved hook appearance
- The separators are placed using aseptic technique and a hand mirror for observation with either a bird beak or #139 pliers
- The clinician grips the short leg of the spring separator with the pliers and positions the long leg under the contact point on the tongue side
- The short leg is released and pulled under the contact point leaving the coil visible on the facial side
- The coil is later used for removal using a scaler by pulling upward while bracing with a finger
- Brass wires are placed by using a hemostat
- They are inserted under the contact from the lingual side and then drawn toward the facial aspect
- The wire ends are twisted together, cut off with a ligature wire cutter, and then inserted close to the gums
- Brass wire separators are removed by cutting them with a ligature cutting pliers and then lifting both parts out on the facial side with a hemostat

ORTHODONTIC BANDS

Posterior orthodontic bands are selected and sized after separators are removed.

- Selection and sizing is done either on the basis of the person's study model or on them directly
- Band size is evaluated further by pressing the band over the occlusal surface with a finger and using a band pusher to seat it onto the tooth and tweak it for fit
- After sizing, the bands are taken off with band removal pliers and put on a model or band block
- The lab technician or orthodontist then readies each band for cementation
- This involves smoothing the surfaces with a bur, a metal tool that removes rough edges
- Pins or wax are put in the openings of bands that will have attached brackets or buccal tubes to keep cement out

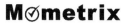

CEMENTED ORTHODONTIC BANDS

Orthodontic band cementation is an example of four-handed dentistry, a cooperative effort between the dentist and assistant.

- Glass ionomer cement, which gives off fluoride, is the most commonly used cement; other choices are zinc phosphate, and polycarboxylate cements
- Aseptic technique and glove use are mandated
- The patient's teeth are polished with a rubber cup, and the mouth is rinsed and dried
- Cotton rolls are used to segregate the areas for band placement
- The assistant mixes the cement, loads the cement onto each band, and hands each to the orthodontist
- There are various band transfer methods such as sequential placement on the mixing slab or use of a spatula, wax or tape
- The assistant provides the band driver and other instruments to the orthodontist as needed
- If the cement becomes too thick, the assistant must clean off instruments using an alcohol wipe or wet gauze and mix more
- Once all bands have been placed, the cement is permitted to set and surplus is removed with a scaler
- Pins or wax, if present, are taken out of the brackets
- The patient's mouth is rinsed at the end
- The assistant is also responsible for clean-up of cement on used instruments

DIRECT BONDING PROCEDURES

After placement of posterior bands is complete, direct bonding of brackets to anterior teeth, generally from the center to the second bicuspids on each side of both arches, is done.

- Aseptic technique and four-handed dentistry are employed
- The patient's teeth are polished with a rubber cup and pumice (not paste), and the person's mouth is rinsed and dried
- The area is segregated using cotton rolls and cheek and lip retractors
- The first step of direct bonding is application of acid etchant to the surface of the enamel per manufacturer's instructions
- The assistant transmits the etchant to the orthodontist for application
- He or she is also responsible for keeping the field dry and later rinsing the etchant off and drying the teeth
- A liquid sealant may then be applied to each surface by the dentist
- The assistant prepares the second ingredient, the bonding agent, spreads it on the back of each bracket, and sequentially transfers brackets to the orthodontist
- The orthodontist uses an orthodontic scaler to remove surplus bonding agent and set and keep the brackets in place until the bonding agent is chemically set or cured with a special light
- Cotton rolls and retractors are removed afterwards

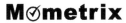

ARCH WIRES AND LIGAMENT TIES PLACEMENT PROCEDURES

Usually, the center of the arch wire is marked and tentatively placed between the central incisors.

- The ends are fit into the buccal tubes of the molar bands with Weingart pliers and then fed through the notches in each bracket
- The Damon St. bracket type has a slot that can be opened up for arch wire positioning and later removal
- Otherwise, placement is done using either elastic ties or ligature wire tires
- Elastomeric ties are placed over each bracket with a hemostat or ligature typing pliers
- Elastic chain ties or rings might also be used
- Ligature wire ties are wrapped around the top and bottom wings of each bracket working toward the midline using a ligature director
- Each tie is twisted together on the mesial side with either a ligature typing pliers or hemostat, and cut about 3 to 5 mm out with ligature wire cutting pliers; the pigtails are tucked under the arch wire toward the gums and interproximal space
- The ties should also be checked for wires sticking out by running a finger along the arch
- Excess arch wire at the distal edges should be removed with distal-end cutting pliers
- Removable rubber elastic bands, if prescribed, are demonstrated and given to the patient

FIXED APPLIANCE PATIENT'S ORAL HYGIENE

Patients with fixed appliances should be supplied with special orthodontic toothbrushes and floss threaders.

- Orthodontic toothbrushes are shaped to maneuver around the brackets and into the area between the gingival margin and the band.
- Teeth are brushed from above the maxillary band or below the mandibular band. Floss is strung through the floss threader and pulled under the arch wire for flossing. Extra time for both brushing and flossing is necessary when a person has a fixed appliance. Fluoride rinses may also be recommended. The patient should be directed to shun foods, such as those that are sticky, brittle or hard, that can damage the appliance parts.

REMOVAL OF FIXED APPLIANCES PROCEDURES

Once the orthodontist feels the patient's teeth have been adequately repositioned, a completion appointment for removal of the fixed appliances is scheduled.

- Ligature ties are taken off first Elastic band ties are released by inserting the end of a scaler explorer through each and pulling them off over the bracket wings
- Ligature wire ties are removed by drawing the twisted portion out from the embrasure, cutting that portion off with a ligature wire cutting pliers, and then pulling each wire out
- The arch wire is taken out using a hemostat to unseat it from each buccal tube
- Anterior brackets are removed by squeezing them between the edges of a bracket and adhesive-removing pliers
- The posterior bands are then taken off with band-removing pliers
- After the buccal side is lifted, the same thing is done on the lingual side until the band comes off

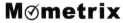

COMPLETION PROCEDURES AFTER REMOVAL OF FIXED APPLIANCES

After fixed appliances are removed, the cement and bonding substances must also be stripped off the tooth surface.

- Devices for this removal include hand scalers, ultrasonic scalers, and finishing burs
- A rubber cup polish is done and photographs may be obtained
- Alginate impressions of both arches are acquired and conveyed to the laboratory for creation of a retainer
- The retainer is usually positioned the same or next day
- Patients should be thoroughly educated on how to put in and take out the retainer and the required wearing schedule
- Sometimes a customized rubber or acrylic positioner might be utilized prior to retainer use
- Retention is important because it supports the teeth against cheek and tongue pressure, restrains additional growth-related changes, and allows healing of gums and periodontal tissues

ULTRASONIC SCALER

Hand scalers generally have straight or curved sickles and pointed tips at each end; they are used most often to remove supragingival calculus.

- An orthodontic scaler is a variant with straighter ends used to direct brackets for placement and remove elastic ties and cement or bonding material
- An alternative for removal of cement and bonding substances (as well as calculus and other deposits) is the ultrasonic scaler
- This machine uses high-frequency sound waves, which it translates into mechanical energy in the form of high-speed vibrations at the tip
- Water also comes out at the tip to control heat buildup
- The combination of vibrational energy and water facilitates thorough removal of debris

DENTAL TREATMENT AREA EQUIPMENT

A comfortable, supportive dental chair with arm support, adjustable headrest, and controls is essential.

- The chair must accommodate upright, supine, and subsupine positions
- There should be ergonomic chairs or stools for both operator and assistant
- It is suggested that the operator's (dentist's) chair be have 5 castors, an adjustable seat and back, and a broad base
- The assistant needs a chair that also has a foot bar for support
- Typically, there is also a track-mounted, iridescent operating light to illuminate the oral cavity
- There should be an air-water syringe to provide streams of water and/or air, an oral evacuation system, and curing light
- The oral evacuation system, which generally includes a saliva ejector and a high velocity evacuation (HVE) device, is part of the overall dental unit, which also includes the air-water syringe and various handpieces
- The curing light is an electronically-controlled blue light-emitting wand that polymerizes resins and composites

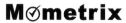

- A foot-controlled rheostat or resistor is also attached to the dental unit and is used for handpiece operation
- If restorations are performed, there is an amalgamator to make the materials

DENTAL OPERATOR AND ASSISTANT SITTING POSITIONS

The dental operator (usually the dentist) should be seated with a straight back, feet planted on the floor, and knees slightly below hip level.

- The chair height should be such that the patient's oral cavity is at the same level as the operator's elbows
- The operator should be relaxed with eyes directed downward toward the patient
- The assistant should be seated about 4 to 5 inches higher than the dentist to permit greater visibility and access
- The patient should also be sitting up straight with the abdominal bar or chair back in a position for support
- An assistant should place his or her feet on the base platform, not the floor, with hips and thighs parallel to the floor at the level of the person's shoulders
- Dental operators are prone to shoulder, neck, and back pain
- Shoulder and neck pain is generally due to extended strain or flexion of the shoulder
- Combined neck and back pain is usually due to prolonged extension or lifting of the arm, and low back pain is most likely due to prolonged bodily twisting
- Carpal tunnel syndrome is another potential injury from repeated wrist flexion and extension

DENTISTRY OPERATING ZONES

Team or four-handed dentistry is usually facilitated by having four distinct zones in the treatment area.

- There is a static zone right behind the patient where the dental unit and possibly a moveable cabinet are located
- The operator's zone is the largest segment
- This is where the operator, the dentist, sits and moves around
- Depending on whether the dentist is right- or left-handed, this zone is either to left or right of the static zone
- The assistant's zone should be directly opposite the operator
- The assistant sits in this area and has a cart with instruments and dental materials
- There is a fourth transfer zone next to the assistant over the region of the patient's chest
- This is the zone where dental materials and instruments are exchanged between assistant and operator
- These zones are often described in terms of parts of the clock

- For a right-handed operator, the static zone is 12 to 2o'clock, and the operator zone is 7 to 12 o'clock; the assistant sits between 2 and 4'oclock and uses 4 to 7 o'clock as the transfer zone

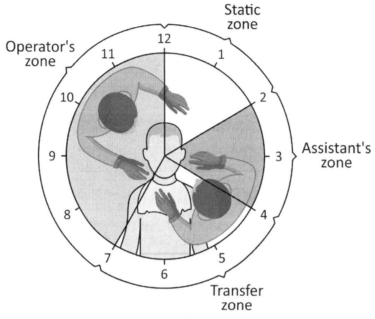

Right-Handed Dentist

INSTRUMENT TRANSFER TECHNIQUES

The assistant should transfer instruments within the transfer zone over the patient's chest.

- Both operator and assistant are gloved
- Instruments should be transferred with as little motion as possible with the working end pointed toward the tooth being worked on and the handle available for grasping by the dentist
- In the single-handed transfer technique, the clinical assistant picks up the instrument from the tray using the thumb and first two fingers of the left hand
- He or she holds the handle end or the side not required
- The instrument is transferred into the transfer zone near the implement in use
- The instruments are exchanged by using the last two fingers of the left hand for retrieval of the used one and folding it into the palm while putting the new tool into the operator's fingers
- The previously used instrument is returned to its correct position in the setup tray
- In the two-handed technique, the new instrument is gripped similarly in the right hand while the used implement is recovered with the left hand and returned to the tray by releasing the palm grasp
- The new instrument is given to the dentist with proper orientation of the working end

UNIQUE INSTRUMENT TRANSFER TECHNIQUES

When initiating a dental procedure, the operator uses the mouth mirror and explorer for examination.

- These should be transferred from the assistant to dentist at the same time using the two-handed technique
- Most instruments are gripped by the dentist in a pen, palm or palm and thumb grasp
- Many of the tools are hinged (pliers, forceps, etc.); in these cases, the assistant should hold the implement at the hinge and put the handle directly into the dentist's palm or over the dentist's fingers
- Transfers using cotton pliers should be done by squeezing the beaks together to avoid dropping the cotton
- Dental materials are transferred much closer to the chin than instruments
- Amalgam can be given to the dentist or, if allowed by state law, directly inserted into the tooth by the dental assistant
- Substances like impression materials and cements that are delivered in syringes can be transferred directly to the dentist with the tip facing the arch on which the dentist is working
- Cements and liners are generally conveyed on mixing slabs along with the applicator device
- The assistant uses the right hand to hold the slab and the left hand to wipe off any excess with gauze

MOUTH RINSING METHODS

The dental assistant is generally responsible for both mouth rinsing and oral evacuation during dental procedures.

- Either a saliva ejector or more powerful high-volume oral evacuator (HVE) can be used for both processes
- Limited-area rinsing is done often during pauses in the procedure to eliminate debris, and a complete mouth rinse should be done at the end
- The assistant grips the air-water syringe in the left hand and the saliva or HVE in the right one
- For a limited rinse, the tip is pointed toward the desired area and air and water are directed to the site; fluid and debris are then suctioned out and the region is dried by compressing the air button
- The patient should be facing the assistant during the final full-mouth rinse, and the HVE or saliva ejector tip should be directed into left part of the oral cavity (without touching tissues)
- The air-water syringe is directed first from right to left along the maxillary arch and then similarly along the mandibular arch
- The suction tip is placed in the back of the mouth to remove the fluid and extracted debris

ORAL EVACUATION METHODS

Moisture control and maintenance of a clinical field are paramount during dental procedures.

- A saliva ejector, a small flexible tube attached to a bulb, is generally used for oral evacuation of minute quantities of saliva or water
- A high-volume oral evacuator (HVE) is usually chosen when more moisture control or removal of debris and other substances such as blood may be needed

- The HVE is essentially a vacuum with a sterile attached tip
- Tips can be made of plastic or stainless steel; they are either straight or slightly angled and are slanted at the working end
- The evacuator should be held by the assistant with either a pen or thumb-to-nose grasp in the same hand as the dentist uses; the assistant then uses his or her other hand for operation of the air-water syringe or for instrument transfer
- The patient's tongue and cheek usually must be isolated from the evacuation site with the HVE tip or the mouth mirror
- There are several techniques for HVE tip placement, including on either the lingual or buccal surface and slightly behind the area being prepared or on the opposite side of the tooth

HIGH-VOLUME EVACUATOR IN POSTERIOR VERSUS ANTERIOR AREAS

When the HVE or high-volume oral evacuator is used in posterior areas, the beveled edge of the tip should be positioned as near to the tooth being prepared as possible and parallel to either the buccal or lingual surface.

- The upper edge of the tip should reach a bit beyond the occlusal surface
- A cotton roll is often placed under the tip for comfort when mandibular areas are being controlled
- For anterior or front teeth, the HVE tip should be positioned parallel to the opposite surface and somewhat beyond the incisal edge of the tooth being prepared
- In other words, lingual and facial preparations require vacuum extraction from the facial and lingual sides respectively

COTTON ROLLS

Cotton rolls are used to isolate and control moisture in a working area during an oral procedure.

- For maxillary placement, the patient faces the assistant with the chin elevated
- Cotton pliers are used to grasp and convey the cotton roll to the mucobuccal fold near the working area of the patient's mouth
- For mandibular placement, the patient faces the assistant with the chin lowered
- The cotton roll is picked up with the cotton pliers and transferred to the corresponding mucobuccal fold
- In this case, another cotton roll is also placed into the floor of the mouth between the operational field and the tongue
- The person may need to raise his or her tongue to facilitate placement
- Cotton rolls used in anterior regions generally need to be bent before positioning
- Rolls should be taken out before the final full-mouth rinse using cotton pliers
- Very dry rolls can stick to the oral mucosa causing tissue damage; in these cases, moistening with water from the air-water syringe is indicated before removal

DRY ANGLES

Dry angles are triangular-shaped absorbent pads that may be used during oral procedures in the back areas of either dental arch.

- The angles are positioned on top of the Stensen's duct on the inside of the cheek near the maxillary second molar
- One type of salivary gland, the parotid gland, leads to the Stensen's duct

82

- Therefore, the main purpose of dry angles is to obstruct the saliva flow into the area
- The pads also preserve the oral tissues
- Dry angles that become saturated with saliva should be replaced
- They should be moistened further with the air-water syringe before removal

DENTAL DAMS

Dental dams are commercially-available barriers that are used to isolate areas during oral procedures.

- They come in latex or latex-free materials in various sizes, colors, and thicknesses
- They are usually divided into sixths with holes punched for placement (explained elsewhere) in the upper or lower middle portion for maxillary or mandibular treatments respectively
- Dental dams are generally utilized for more involved procedures requiring local anesthesia
- A dental dam provides area infection and moisture control
- It inhibits contact with debris and dental materials
- The patient is less likely to accidentally inhale or swallow materials
- The dam aids the dentist and assistant through improved access because it retracts the lips, tongue, and gums
- It also enhances visibility of the area by providing color contrast
- In some states, the dental assistant may legally place the dental dam

DENTAL DAM EQUIPMENT

The dental dam is held in a dental dam frame, which is a three-sided plastic or metal used to position the dam.

- A dental dam napkin is a cotton sheet that is put between the dam and patient to absorb moisture
- A dental dam punch is a specialized type of hole puncher that is used to make holes in the dental dam where the teeth to be worked on are isolated
- Punches come in 5 sizes depending on the type of tooth involved: Nos. 1 and 2 for mandibular and maxillary incisors respectively, No. 3 for canines and premolars, No. 4 for molars and bridge abutments, and No. 5 (the largest) for the anchor tooth
- The anchor tooth is the one chosen to hold the dental dam clamp, thus, securing the dam
- Dental dam clamps are generally made of stainless steel in the shape of the crown; they come in cervical, winged, and wingless conformations and have a bow, jaws, and forceps holes
- Dental dam forceps are utilized for dam positioning and removal
- Lubricant and a dental dam stamp are also necessary
- The latter is an ink-pad stamp made like a dental arch that serves as a guide to indicate teeth to be punched out on the dam

DENTAL DAM PREPARATION

Local anesthetic is administered first by the dentist with help from the assistant.

- It is important to note any misaligned or malpositioned teeth at this time because if a tooth is not in the correct position, holes must be punched in a different spot in the dam
- The width of the arch should also be noted for possible accommodations
- The assistant then applies lubricant to the person's lip with a cotton roll or applicator

- The location of potential dam placement is inspected with a mouth mirror and explorer
- If there is any debris or plaque in the area, certain teeth should be brushed or coronally polished prior to dam positioning
- All regional contacts should be flossed to avoid tearing the dam
- A dental dam stamp is marked to identify the teeth for isolation in a particular arch
- Using this template, the dental dam is punched with the dam punch with the holes for the anchor and the tooth for isolation
- It is essential to use the correct size punch
- Holes going over tight contacts should be lubricated with water-soluble lubricant on the underside

PLACEMENT OF A DENTAL DAM

The correct clamp is attached to both a floss safety line and locked dental dam forceps.

- It is fit over the anchor tooth by initial placement over the lingual side followed by widening of the forceps and positioning the buccal side
- The previously punched dental dam is placed over the clamp bow using the index fingers to stretch it over the clamp and anchor tooth
- The safety line should also be pulled to the outside
- The dam is fastened to the last tooth at the opposite end with floss or some type of cord
- Then, the dental napkin is placed between the outer parts of the dam and the patient's mouth
- The dental dam frame is affixed over the oral cavity to hold the dam in place
- The other teeth are then isolated through the punched holes and pushed into place using dental floss or tape
- The teeth are dried with the air syringe
- All edges must be sealed by tucking or inverting them into the sulcus of the gum using some type of tucking instrument before performing the desired procedure

REMOVAL OF A DENTAL DAM

The first step of dental dam removal is stretching of the dam material outward with the middle or index finger and cutting each interseptal dam.

- The dam clamp is taken off with the dam forceps by placing them into the forceps holes and compressing the handles to open the jaws of the clamp
- The clamp may need to be rotated toward each side for removal
- The holder, dam material and napkin are removed
- The dam is examined to make sure no material is left interdentally, and flossing is done if indicated
- The gum around the anchor tooth is kneaded to improve circulation
- The individual's mouth is rinsed and debris is removed

CORONAL POLISH

A coronal polish is a process by which soft deposits and extrinsic stains are removed from the clinical crown of teeth.

- An abrasive material is used
- A dental handpiece and a rubber cup are generally utilized for application but brushes, dental tape, or floss are sometimes substituted

- Coronal polishing is usually done after hard deposits have been scaled off
- There are several reasons the procedure is performed. It helps the patient maintain clean teeth and sustain good oral hygiene
- The procedure enhances fluoride absorption and discourages buildup of new deposits
- In terms of dental processes, coronal polishing is used to prepare teeth for use of enamel sealant and for positioning of orthodontic brackets and bands
- In many states, the dental assistant or hygienist can legally perform a coronal polish instead of the dentist in which case the assistant is seated in the appropriate operator position

MATERIALS THAT CAN/CANNOT BE REMOVED BY CORONAL POLISH

A coronal polish can remove soft deposits and extrinsic stains.

- Calculus, hard calcified deposits, and intrinsic stains are generally not eliminated through coronal polishing
- Calculus is removed prior to the polish via scaling
- Intrinsic stains within the tooth structure are usually permanent; they include dental fluorosis and stains contracted through metal or tetracycline exposure or pulp damage
- There are four types of soft deposits removed by coronal polishing
- Two of these, materia alba and plaque, contain microorganisms
- Materia alba is a less structured precursor to plaque development, which can lead to tooth decay, gingivitis, and periodontal disease
- The other types of soft deposits are food debris and pellicle, which is a thin film containing saliva and sulcular fluid
- Extrinsic stains from endogenous sources can be removed by coronal polishing as well and include stains associated with poor dental hygiene (yellow or brown), tobacco stains, and others

ABRASIVE USE

Abrasives are particulate materials that create friction and roughness to smooth out the tooth surface during coronal polishing.

- They come in powder or paste form and usually also contain water, a binder, a humectant for water retention, coloring, and flavoring
- Available abrasive agents include fluoride pastes, flour of pumice, chalk, zirconium silicate, and tin oxide
- The rate of abrasion for a particular type of abrasive is dependent upon the characteristics of the abrasive material, the speed of the handpiece, the pressure and amount applied, and the moisture level
- Abrasiveness is increased if the particles are sharp-edged, firmer, stronger, larger in size, or resist becoming embedded in the tooth surface

RUBBER PROPHY CUP

Rubber prophy cups are formulated with natural or synthetic rubber.

- They are attached at an angle to a low-speed dental handpiece for coronal polishing
- Sometimes a disclosing agent for easier recognition of plaque is applied to tooth surfaces before polishing (and perhaps at the end for checking) with a cotton tip applicator
- An abrasive agent is placed into the cup
- Note that if more than one type of abrasive is used for the polishing, individual cups are used for each

85

- A modified pen grasp is generally used to hold the handpiece with cup, and speed is regulated by foot pressure on the rheostat
- One quadrant is usually done at a time
- The operator starts the polishing by positioning the cup near the sulcus of the gum on the mesial or distal surface of a tooth
- He or she employs gentle pressure to bend the cup working toward the occlusal or incisal edge
- The cup is lifted a bit, and the procedure is duplicated on the other side of the tooth
- The operator then repeats the same process on the adjacent tooth and so on
- Frequent rinsing and removal of debris is suggested during the procedure and at the end

PROPHY BRUSH

Prophy brushes are soft, supple brushes made of nylon or natural bristles.

- They are attached to a low-speed dental handpiece and are used to polish only the enamel surfaces of teeth (that is, no contact with the gums)
- This procedure is done after the rubber cup polish. Prophy paste is spread over the brush
- The polishing starts with the most posterior tooth to be done
- For the back teeth, the major objective is the polishing of the occlusal surfaces
- For each posterior tooth, the brush is directed from the central fossa first toward the mesial buccal cusp tip and then toward the distal buccal cusp
- For the anterior teeth, the brush is positioned in the lingual pit above the cingulum and then directed toward the incisal edge during polishing
- All lingual surfaces with pits or grooves should be polished similarly
- At the end, the mouth is rinsed and cleared of debris

DENTAL TAPE OR DENTAL FLOSS

After teeth have undergone a coronal polish using a prophy cup and a prophy brush, they should be polished further using dental tape and floss.

- Both are used interproximally
- A 12 to 18 inch piece of dental tape is utilized first
- An abrasive is applied to the interproximal contact places between teeth using a finger or a cotton tip applicator
- One quadrant is usually done at a time
- The dental tape is manipulated between the middle fingers of each hand
- It is inserted obliquely into the contact area using a back-and-forth motion and light pressure and then wrapped around the tooth
- The proximal surfaces of each tooth are polished with the tape moving along adjacent teeth
- The mouth is rinsed and evacuated
- Any remaining residue is then removed by using dental floss and subsequent rinsing
- Unwaxed floss should be used if fluoride application is to be done afterwards because waxed floss coats the teeth and deters fluoride absorption

SUPPLEMENTAL EQUIPMENT

A good dental light and mouth mirror are needed.

- Cheek retractors are usually necessary at some point
- Oral cavity maintenance using the air-water syringe, evacuator, saliva ejector, and possibly wipes is essential
- There are a number of supplementary polishing aids that might be utilized during the final phase in conjunction with dental tape and floss
- One aid that is useful for people with orthodontic work is a bridge threader
- A bridge threader is a plastic piece with a loop through which dental tape or floss can be threaded to work around orthodontic or other appliances
- There are also various grit size abrasive polishing strips that can be employed on enamel facades and soft wood points that can be used with abrasives
- Small interproximal brushes can be utilized for navigation around orthodontic appliances and other contact areas

DENTAL PLAQUE

Dental plaque is a tacky, bacteria-containing mass found on teeth that have not been brushed thoroughly.

- It looks like a soft, white, sticky accumulation and is often found in areas near the gingival
- The bacteria feed off consumed sugar and convert it to acid
- The acid in turn damages the tooth enamel by causing a process called demineralization
- The content of the minerals calcium and phosphate is depressed
- Demineralization on enamel surfaces looks chalky and white
- This is often a problem found in patients who have had orthodontic appliances removed where the brackets were previously situated
- Eventually plaque that has not been removed can lead to tooth decay

DISCLOSING AGENTS

Disclosing agents are impermanent coloring agents (usually red) that adhere to and visualize plaque.

- They come in various chewable tablet and liquid forms
- The latter can be painted onto the teeth or put on the tongue
- Disclosing agents can be used to encourage good oral hygiene by showing the patient areas of plaque
- They are often also used as part of a coronal polishing procedure
- The dental assistant or hygienist may do disclosing agent application in the office
- He or she should wear personal protective equipment (PPE) during the procedure
- As preparation, petroleum jelly is spread over the lips and tooth-colored restorations
- If the disclosing agent is in liquid form, the operator applies it to the surface of teeth using a cotton tip applicator and a dappen dish
- If tablets are used, the individual chews the tablet and swirls it around in the mouth
- Excess solution is rinsed and withdrawn
- Plaque is visualized by the patient with a hand mirror and the operator with a mouth mirror
- The plaque present is then charted by the operator using an overglove
- Patient education about oral hygiene should be the last step

FLUORIDE

Fluoride is a mineral derivative of element fluorine.

- It is primarily absorbed via the gastrointestinal tract and is found in low amounts in normal bone and dental enamel
- Average fluoride levels are lower in teeth with caries
- Fluoride incorporated into tooth enamel forms fluoroapatite crystals
- If high amounts are ingested during tooth development, teeth can acquire a mottled appearance known as fluorosis
- Excessive amounts of fluoride can cause toxicity in the form of chronic or rarely acute fluoride poisoning
- Chronic fluoride poisoning from habitual ingestion (such as in areas of fluoridation of the water supply) can cause the mottled appearance (~up to 1.8 ppm) or enamel hypocalcification (~1.8 to 2.0 ppm)
- The latter changes the enamel structure and manifests as chalky or discolored bands and flecks, cracks, and pits
- Optimal fluoride exposure should be between 0.7 and 1.2 ppm giving the teeth a gleaming, white, unblemished appearance

FLUORIDE BENEFITS

Fluoride has beneficial effects, primarily the reduction of dental caries, because it binds to the bacteria in plaque, thus, retarding acid production and decay.

- Therefore, fluoride is often administered systemically or topically
- Systemic sources of fluoride include fluoridation of the water supply (usually in the form of sodium fluoride), ingestion of foods containing fluoride (like meat, cereals, and citrus fruits), or in the form of prescribed tablets, drops, or special vitamin preparations
- The latter are usually given to children up until their second molar erupts
- Fluoride can also be applied topically in the form of sodium fluoride, stannous fluoride, or acidulated phosphate fluoride
- Topical fluoride only accesses the outer enamel layer
- Dentifrices (toothpastes) and polishing pastes usually contain fluoride for topical application
- Children should also get special topical application of fluoride in the dental office once or twice yearly to reduce decay

FLUORIDE CHOICES

Topical fluoride application in the dental office is usually done using 2% sodium fluoride, 8% stannous fluoride, or 1.23% acidulated phosphate fluoride (APF).

- The sodium fluoride preparations are stable, do not cause discoloration, and are gentle to tissues, but they must be applied weekly for 4 weeks each time
- The stannous fluoride has many disadvantages, including instability, a caustic taste, and discoloration due to tin in the preparation
- Thus, the APF preparations are used most often as they are non-irritating, have a mild taste, do not cause discoloration, and need to be used only once or twice a year
- APF preparations should be kept in plastic containers to discourage acidification

FLUORIDE PROCEDURES

The dental assistant performs the procedure after a rubber cup polish.

- Application should never be done before placement of orthodontic bands or sealants as it deters adhesion
- The assistant dons personal protective equipment
- Fluoride trays that encompass all erupted teeth but do not extend beyond them are selected
- About a third of each tray is filled with the fluoride gel or foam
- Teeth are dried with the air syringe and then the tray(s) is (are) positioned
- The trays should be shifted up and down to distribute the fluoride preparation
- Saliva and moisture is removed using the saliva ejector, which is kept inserted with the patient's mouth closed for the time specified for the preparation
- The ejector and trays are then removed and the mouth is evacuated
- The patient should be advised not to eat, drink, or rinse for a half hour after application
- Using overgloves, the dental assistant charts the application and any consequences
- An alternative to foam or gel application is the use of a fluoride rinse after tooth brushing or a rubber cup polish

EXTRAORAL HEADGEAR

Extraoral headgear is one type of removable orthodontic appliance.

- It is designed to be worn several hours a day in conjunction with intraoral orthodontic appliances, for application of force to move teeth, or for modification of cranial-facial bone growth
- There are many designs for extra oral headgear, but in general, there are two portions
- One part is the facebow which is usually attached to the buccal tubes on the maxillary first molars
- The facebow's main function is the creation of more room in the arch by either stabilizing or actually moving the molar distally
- A traction device is connected to the outer part of the facebow for application of extraoral force
- This traction device is usually some sort of adjustable strap that goes around the head
- The possible configurations for a traction device include a high-pull, cervical, chin cap, or combination type

RETRACTORS AND MOUTH PROPS

Retractors are utilized to redirect tissue in order to perform certain procedures.

- They are often used in oral surgery but have other applications
- There are tissue, cheek and lip, and tongue retractors
- Tissue retractors have small jagged edges on the working end to grasp tissue, and usually look like forceps or cotton pliers
- Cheek and lip retractors are large metal or plastic apparatuses that fit into the mouth to pull the cheeks or lips outward expanding the viewing region
- Tongue retractors are spoon-shaped or lengthy blades that are used to displace the tongue
- They are designed to be put between the rim of the tongue and the lingual surfaces of the teeth
- They can also be used for cheek retraction by positioning them on the buccal mucosa

- Hemostats or needle holders, which are both forceps with jagged beaks and locking handles, may be used for retraction as well
- Mouth props are devices that are inserted for longer periods of time when necessary to keep the patient's mouth open
- They may be constructed of stainless steel, silicone, plastic, or hard rubber, and come in various sizes
- The locking Molt mouth gag is an example

PSYCHOLOGY

Psychology is the study of the mind and people's characteristic mental makeup.

- Everyone brings an acquired belief system or paradigm to his or her interactions with others
- Patients all have certain preconceived ideas about dental practices

COMMUNICATION AND LISTENING SKILLS

Successful patient interaction and management can be facilitated by understanding people's paradigms and use of good communication and listening skills

- Communication is the exchange of information
- Good communication consists of skillful interpretation of the message by the sender (in this case the dental professional), interpretation of the message by the receiver (the patient), and establishment of a connection as indicated by feedback
- Active listening on the part of both sender and receiver enhances good communication

VERBAL AND NONVERBAL COMMUNICATION

Any type of communication between people that does not involve words is nonverbal communication, which probably plays a larger role in the interaction than verbalization.

- This is particularly true in a dental office where patients may not be able to speak during a procedure or may have apprehensions
- Patient responses can be indicated by nonverbal cues, such as facial expressions, gestures, or posture and position
- Patient resistance is suggested by a tight posture and/or crossed arms and legs
- Conversely, patient openness is indicated by a relaxed posture and uncrossed appendages
- The posture of the dental assistant can affect the patient as well; generally sitting close to the patient is better than towering over the patient
- The dental professional should also be sure that he or she maintains the proper spatial distance from the patient
- Patients generally feel more comfortable when they have been well-informed beforehand and the professional works from the side

MULTI-CULTURAL COMMUNICATION

Various cultures have different value systems.

- The dental professional needs to be aware of these different systems in dealing with patients
- This is particularly true in this day and age in the United States with such a large, expanding, and diverse immigrant population

- For example, eye contact between individuals or use of first names versus surnames differs among cultures
- One of the most important considerations is whether or not the patient whose first language is not English fully understands information
- This can be facilitated by speaking slowly, facing the individual while talking, using a translator, and getting more than perfunctory feedback from the patient during the communication

PAIN TYPES AND ANXIETY

Before, during, and/or after dental procedures, some type of pain and anxiety control may need to be administered to the patient.

- Pain and anxiety can be alleviated through psychological methods or various chemical or physiologic agents
- The latter generally fall into 5 categories: local or topical anesthesia, inhalation sedation, antianxiety drugs, intravenous sedation, or general anesthesia
- An anesthetic is a substance that dulls pain and, in some cases, induces unconsciousness
- A sedative is a tranquilizing agent that induces a state of calm and drowsiness
- Antianxiety agents are drugs that relieve apprehension

TOPICAL AND LOCAL ANESTHETICS

All anesthetics block nerve impulses, thus, dulling pain sensations.

- Topical anesthetics are spread directly over oral mucosa areas, generally before application of a local anesthetic agent
- Topical preparations usually come in ointment form and are applied with a cotton-tip applicator, but they also come as sprays, liquids, and patches
- Local anesthetics come in the form of chemical amides and esters and are generally injected in the proximity of the nerve associated with the tooth being treated
- Local anesthetic agents have a particular time frame after injection for induction of full numbing and later loss of numbing (duration)
- Local anesthetics are classified in terms of their duration as short-, intermediate- or long-acting. Most procedures require the intermediate-acting duration of 2 to 4 hours
- Most intermediate- and long-acting local anesthetic agents also contain small concentrations of vasoconstrictors, such as epinephrine, which decrease blood flow and bleeding to the region
- These preparations may be contraindicated in patients with hypertension, cardiovascular disease, liver or kidney disease, hyperthyroidism
- These drugs may also be contraindicated for patients who are pregnant

LOCAL ANESTHESIA

Local anesthesia methods fall into 3 main categories: local infiltration, field block, and nerve block.

- Local infiltration anesthesia involves injection of the agent into gingival tissues near the small terminal nerve branches, numbing the necessary tooth and/or gums. The anesthetic can also be injected using pressure right into the periodontal ligament

- With field block anesthesia, the agent is injected close to the larger terminal nerve limbs near the apex of the tooth. The advantages of this technique are avoidance of messages to the central nervous system and swiftness of action
- In nerve block anesthesia, the agent is introduced close to a main nerve trunk, which eliminates pain sensations to the brain and over a relatively large local area

MAXILLARY LOCAL ANESTHESIA INJECTION SITES

Local infiltration or field block techniques are used to desensitize individual maxillary teeth by injecting near the apex of specific anterior teeth.

- Various nerve blocks are used to numb certain teeth or areas
- A nasopalatine nerve block, in which the lingual tissue next to the incisive papilla is injected, numbs the front of the hard palate between the canines
- The greater palatine nerve block uses injection near the second molar and in front of the greater palatine foramen to block sensations to the entire hard palate and soft tissues posterior to the canine
- A maxillary nerve block is done by introducing the anesthetic into the mucobuccal fold near the second molar, which blocks one entire oral quadrant as well as skin on that side of the nose, cheek, upper lip, and lower eyelid
- The anterior superior alveolar, middle superior alveolar, and posterior superior alveolar nerve blocks involve injection into the fold at the first premolar, the fold at the second premolar, and near the apex of the second molar respectively; each affects 2 to 3 close teeth (and tissues for the last)

MANDIBULAR LOCAL ANESTHESIA INJECTION SITES

Local infiltration (or field block techniques) are used to desensitize individual mandibular teeth by injecting near the apex of specific anterior teeth.

- Nerve blocks are used to numb larger areas. Introduction into the mucobuccal fold in front of the mental foramen is known as an incisive nerve block; it affects teeth from the central incisors back to the premolars plus buccal tissues in the area
- The inferior alveolar nerve block or mandibular block dulls an entire quadrant including teeth, mucous membranes, the front portion of the tongue and mouth floor, plus soft tissues; it involves injection into the mandibular ramus behind the retromolar pad
- The lingual nerve block, in which the anesthetic is introduced lingually to the mandibular ramus and next to the maxillary tuberosity, affects the mandibular teeth, the side of the tongue, and lingual tissues on one side
- Other nerve blocks include the buccal nerve block in which the agent is injected into the mucous membrane behind the last available molar just to numb buccal tissue; and the mental nerve block injected between the apices of the premolars to target the premolars, canines, and close facial tissues

ANESTHETIC SYRINGE

An anesthetic or aspirating syringe consists of the anesthetic syringe, disposable needle, and anesthetic cartridge.

- Both reusable stainless steel and disposable plastic syringes may be used
- The syringe portion has a thumb ring for the operator's thumb at one end and a finger grip and bar below it to brace the index and middle fingers during administration

- The barrel of the syringe is a long shaft open on one side for cartridge insertion with a window for observation on the other side
- Inside the barrel is a plunger or piston rod attached to a barbed-tipped harpoon at its end
- There is a threaded tip at the end of the syringe to which the sterile disposable needle is attached
- The needle has a short cartridge end attached to needle hub which is either pushed or screwed onto the threaded tip of the syringe
- The slanted tip on the other end used for tissue penetration is the bevel; the segment between is the shank with its internal, hollow lumen through which the solution travels
- Anesthetic cartridges containing the agent are made of glass
- They have a rubber stopper end to attach to the harpoon of the syringe and an aluminum cap end for needle insertion

CODING ANESTHETIC CARTRIDGES

Anesthetic cartridges conforming to the American Dental Association's seal of acceptance utilize standardized color codes on a band near the rubber stopper end of the cartridge.

- Sometimes the aluminum cap is also colored similarly, although it may be silver
- There is unambiguous, black lettering on the cartridge identifying the agent and concentration
- Some other cartridges have colored writing on the side
- The ADA-approved color schemes are as follows:
  - Articaine 4% with epinephrine 1:100,000 - gold
  - Bupicaine with epinephrine - blue
  - Lidocaine 2% either plain or with epinephrine 1:50,000 or1:100,000 - light blue, green, or red respectively
  - Mepivacaine 3% or 2% with levonordefrin 1:20,000 - tan or brown respectively
  - Prilocaine 4% without or with epinephrine 1:200,000 - black or yellow respectively

ASPIRATING SYRINGE HANDLING

The harpoon of a stainless-steel reusable aspirating syringe should be cleaned after each use and the entire syringe should be autoclaved.

- From time to time, parts should be lubricated or the harpoon may need to be exchanged
- Plastic syringes should be discarded
- The dental needle should be discarded into a sharps container after normal use if there is any evidence of a broken seal, or if tissue penetration occurs more than about 4 times
- Anesthetic cartridges come in sterilized sealed blister packs and should be stored at room temperature in a dark area
- They must be inspected before use and discarded if they are expired or have large bubbles, rust, corrosion, or extruded stoppers
- They are discarded after use

ANESTHETIC SYRINGE PREP

The dental assistant is generally responsible for preparation of the anesthetic syringe outside the viewing area of the patient.

- The sterile syringe is taken out of the autoclave pouch
- While holding the syringe in the left hand, the assistant withdraws the piston rod using the thumb ring
- The rubber stopper end of the cartridge is positioned with the right hand into the barrel of the syringe
- The harpoon is connected to the rubber stopper using medium pressure on the finger ring
- The cap of the syringe end of the disposable needle is taken off and screwed or pushed onto the threaded tip of the syringe
- The assistant removes the needle guard and checks for operation by forcing out a small amount of reagent while holding the syringe upright

TOPICAL AND LOCAL ANESTHETICS ASSISTANCE

The topical anesthetic is applied by drying the area with a sterile gauze sponge and placing the topical preparation on the injection site with a cotton-tip applicator for about a minute.

- The assistant prepares the local anesthetic (as described elsewhere)
- He or she transfers the syringe to the dentist either beneath the patient's chin or behind the patient's head
- The syringe should passed with the thumb ring toward the dentist , the bevel of the needle facing the alveolar bone, and the protective cap secure but loose enough to remove during the transfer
- The dentist does the injection, but the assistant should be observing the patient for any untoward reactions
- The operator then replaces the needle guard with a scooping technique or a mechanical recapping device
- If further anesthesia is needed, the assistant swaps in a new cartridge and transfers it as above
- The recapped syringe is put on the tray
- At the end, the patient's mouth is rinsed and evacuated
- The needle (with the cap) is removed by unscrewing or cutting it off and discarding it in the sharps container
- The cartridge is removed by retraction of the piston and deposited in medical waste
- The syringe should be sterilized

ALTERNATIVE METHODS OF LOCAL ANESTHETICS

One relatively painless and fast method is intraosseous anesthesia in which the cortical plate of bone is first perforated using a solid needle connected to a slow handpiece.

- The anesthetic agent is then injected into the hole using an 8 mm, 27-gauge needle
- Periodontal ligament injection entails insertion into the gingival sulcus
- A special injection syringe is used; it is gun-like in appearance and the syringe is attached externally
- Another technique is intrapulpal injection right into the pulp chamber or root canal using a 25- or 27-gauge needle

- There are computer operated delivery systems available for administration of local anesthesia
- They offer the ability to control parameters such as rate of delivery and pressure
- There are also systems that deliver electronic impulses instead of chemical preparations in cases where the latter are contraindicated

NITROUS OXIDE SEDATION

Nitrous oxide (N_2O) and oxygen (O_2) gases are dispensed simultaneously to a patient through a small nosepiece connected via tubing to a tank.

- The inhaled gases migrate through the nasopharynx through the respiratory chambers eventually reaching the alveoli in the lungs
- The gasses are exchanged between the alveoli and the blood plasma and red cells
- They gases being transported by the blood travel in the circulatory system to the brain, where the analgesic effect is initiated
- Analgesics are agents that relieve pain without loss of consciousness
- Nitrous oxide and oxygen together have mild pharmacologic activity in the central nervous system
- They create a state of calmness for the patient or sedation
- The setup generally includes an inside mask for inhalation of the gases and an outer mask attached to an external reservoir bag and vacuum to carry away exhaled and excess gas

NITROUS OXIDE SAFETY

The American Dental Association suggests that personnel in dental offices utilizing nitrous oxide be monitored twice a year using dosimetry or infrared spectrophotometry.

- Nitrous oxide sedation should not be used with certain patient groups
- Since nitrous oxide has been associated with infertility problems, these include pregnant women in their first trimester and infertile individuals undergoing in-vitro fertilization procedures
- Nitrous oxide is also contraindicated in patients with neurological issues, people with drug abuse problems, those undergoing psychiatric treatment, immunocompromised patients in danger of bone marrow suppression, or people who cannot nose breathe
- On the other hand, nitrous oxide use is a good choice for apprehensive patients, those with sensitive gag reflexes, people who can effectively nose breathe, or individuals with heart conditions
- The latter group benefits from the oxygen administration and reduction of stress

DISPENSATION AND MONITORING

Depending on the state, these functions may be done by the dental assistant under supervision of the dentist or as a cooperative effort.

- The assistant is responsible for rechecking equipment, monitoring gas levels in the tanks, and preparing the patient
- The latter includes explaining the procedures and hazards involved and obtaining informed consent from the individual
- The patient should be lying back. A sterile nitrous mask is attached to the tubing connected to the tanks and then placed over the patient's nose
- The patient is told to breathe slowly through the nose

- When indicated by the dentist, oxygen alone is initially administered for about a minute at a rate of at least 5 liters per minute to determine the normal tidal volume
- Then, nitrous oxide is administered in 500 ml to 1 liter increments a minute with equivalent reduction of oxygen flow
- Patient response is observed by the assistant to determine the optimal mixture that provides sedation without impeding cognition
- The local anesthetic is given a few minutes after nitrous oxide administration is initiated

RECOVERY PROCEDURES

When the dental procedure is almost finished, recovery from nitrous oxide sedation should be initiated.

- The first step is to turn off the nitrous oxide under the dentist's direction
- This oxygenation step allows the patient to receive only oxygen for about 5 minutes to stave off diffusion hypoxia, the inadequate supply of oxygen to bodily tissues
- The patient's mask is then removed and he or she should be brought upright to avoid postural hypotension or fainting
- The patient should not be allowed to go until he or she feels clear- headed (usually a few minutes)
- Nitrous oxide administration, including baseline levels of both gases and the patient's reactions, should be noted on the patient's chart
- The connecting tubing should be disinfected
- Depending on office procedures, the masks may be discarded or given to the patient for later reuse

Chairside Materials

BITING FORCES

Anything that exerts a push or pull on an object is a force.

- The object, in turn, resists the force causing stress
- Significant stress can cause a strain or alteration in the object
- There are three forms of stress and strain that can occur
- All of these types of stress and strain apply to dentistry and need to be considered when selecting dental materials because biting forces are significant
- People bite down on molars with forces in the range of 130 to 170 pounds and about a quarter of that on incisors
  - The first type of stress and strain is tensile force or outward stretching and pulling, which can cause elongation. Elastic bands used in orthodontics can cause tensile stress and strain
  - Another category is compressive force, or pushing together, which occurs during chewing or biting. It is important to select dental materials that can withstand tensile and compressive forces, properties known as ductility and malleability respectively
  - The last type of force to consider is shearing. This occurs when teeth slide across one another from side to side, such as when people grind their teeth (bruxism)

ACIDITY

The parameter pH is a measurement of the relative acidity, neutrality, or alkalinity of a solution or environment.

- It is quantified on a scale from 0 to 14 with low numbers indicating acidic environments, a pH of 7.0 indicating neutrality, and high numbers indicating alkalinity
- Normally, the oral cavity is maintained at relative neutrality by saliva, but certain foods and bacteria are acidic, causing ongoing fluctuations in pH
- Dental materials must be selected to withstand these fluctuations
- Some dental materials themselves are acidic, potentially damaging gum tissues or pulp. If used, these materials must be set up and inserted cautiously

DENTAL MATERIALS THERMAL PROPERTIES

The important thermal properties of a potential dental material are its thermal conductivity and its thermal expansion.

- Thermal conductivity refers to the facility to convey heat
- Materials with lower thermal conductivity are preferred, particularly if they are to be used near the dental pulp
- Thermal expansion refers to the rate of expansion and contraction when exposed to temperature variations
- It is important to select a material that has thermal expansion rates similar to that of tooth structure
- Thermal expansion can cause dimensional changes in the dental material, particularly during the setting process
- This can result in a phenomenon called microleakage in which debris and saliva leak into the area between the tooth and restorative material
- Later tooth sensitivity or caries can result

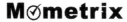

DENTISTRY RETENTION

Retention is the act of keeping or holding something in place.

- In dentistry, retention is achieved by either mechanical or chemical means
- Dental materials are held in place by mechanical retention by slanting the cavity walls inward, abrading the tooth surface with an etchant, or furrowing the cavity walls
- Chemical retention is achieved by some sort of chemical reaction between the dental material and the tooth surface
- If is often used for insertion of gold inlays or crowns which must be indirectly retained through use of cements or bonding agents

PROPERTIES OF DENTAL MATERIALS

Some important properties of dental materials to consider before selection include the following:

1. Adhesion - the ability of dissimilar materials to stick together, either chemically or physically
2. Elasticity - the capacity to undergo distortion and return to the original conformation such as rubber bands within their elastic limit
3. Flow - gradual continual shape change under force such as compression-associated amalgam changes
4. Hardness - relative ability to resist scratching or denting
5. Solubility - capacity to dissolve in fluid; extremely soluble materials are undesirable if in contact with saliva
6. Viscosity - thickness or facility of a liquid to flow
7. Wettability - the capacity of a liquid (the dental material) to flow over and sink into another material (the tooth)
8. Corrosiveness - the ability to react with food or saliva causing pitting, coarseness, or tarnishing with metal-containing materials
9. Galvanism - electric shock caused by reaction between dissimilar metals and carried by saliva

CEMENTS CATEGORIES

Dental cements are agents that bond other dental materials like restorations to the teeth.

- They come in various forms that generally require mixing and preparation before use
- The cements are hardened either by chemical self-curing or light curing with a special light
- They are defined as temporary, intermediate, or permanent cements, depending on the expected duration
- There are also thin liners that are used to seal and protect the pulp or wall and floor of the cavity
- Bases are relatively strong dental cements that are thickly spread in layer between the tooth and restoration for pulp protection
- Besides restorations, cements are also utilized as luting or bonding agents to apply things such as orthodontic bands, bridges, or inlays to the teeth

DENTAL CEMENTS TYPES

Most dental cements are permanent cements.

- These include zinc phosphate, reinforced zinc oxide eugenol, polycarboxylate, glass ionomer, resin cement, resin-reinforced glass ionomer, and compomers
- The cements that are used for permanent cementation of orthodontic bands and brackets are zinc phosphate, polycarboxylate, glass ionomer, and resin cement
- These are all bases and are also used to cement crowns, inlays, onlays, and bridges
- Glass ionomer is also utilized to seal root canals and for restorations
- Reinforced zinc oxide eugenol is generally not used for orthodontic work
- Resin cement is also employed for cementation of enzootic posts, ceramic or composite inlays and onlays, and resin-bonded bridges
- Compomers are resins altered with polyacid
- Resin-reinforced glass ionomer is generally used for metallic or porcelain-fused metallic restorations
- Zinc oxide eugenol is generally used for temporary cementation of crowns, inlays, onlays, and bridges
- It is also used as a root canal sealant or as a periodontal dressing after surgery
- Varnish and calcium hydroxide are examples of liners

ZINC PHOSPHATE CEMENTS

Zinc oxide cement preparations are composed of two parts that are mixed together.

- The first is powder made of zinc oxide plus a small quantity of magnesium oxide and tints of white, yellow, or gray
- The second part is buffered phosphoric acid solution
- When the two are combined, a heat-liberating or exothermic reaction occurs, which must be dampened during preparation using a cooled glass slab and spatula
- The mixture hardens within about 5 minutes and is very strong
- The mechanism of bonding is mechanical interlocking
- The desired consistency depends on the use; it should be creamy in texture for luting and similar to thick putty for use as a base

ZINC PHOSPHATE CEMENT MIXING

The dental or orthodontic assistant mixes the zinc phosphate cement on a clean, cooled glass slab.

- The powder portion is spread and flattened and divided with a stainless-steel cement spatula on one end of the slab
- The liquid portion is dispensed with the dropper bottle unto the other end
- The flat side of the spatula is used to integrate a portion of the powder into the liquid for about 15 seconds
- The mixture is spread over a larger area of the slab and slowly more powder is mixed in with the spatula until the desired thickness is achieved
- The mass is formed into a ball and transferred to the dentist on the slab under the person's chin
- The assistant also transfers a plastic filling instrument to the dentist
- The slab and spatula are wiped with moistened gauze, soaked in water or bicarbonate, and then sterilized or disinfected

ZOE CEMENTS

Zinc oxide eugenol (ZOE) cement comes in two types.

- The traditional type I preparation consists of a powder containing zinc oxide, zinc acetate, resin, and an accelerator, which are mixed with the liquid eugenol
- It is generally used only for temporary cementation or for applications such as post-surgical periodontal dressing because of its soothing properties
- The variant type II preparation is reinforced with alumina and other resins and alumina in the powder and ethoxybenzoic acid in the eugenol, and it is useful for up to a year as an intermediate restorative material (IRM)
- Zinc oxide eugenol is very soluble and of neutral pH
- When reinforced, ZOE is also fairly strong
- ZOE is incompatible with acrylic or composite restorations
- Mixing is done on either a paper pad or glass slab using a stainless-steel cement spatula
- Eugenol disintegrates rubber so it should not come in contact with bulb causing contamination
- ZOE preparations are generally not used for orthodontic procedures

ZOE CEMENT MIXING PROCEDURES

These procedures are done by the dental assistant.

- For powder/liquid systems, the powder is dispensed onto the mixing pad (paper or glass) followed by the liquid
- The two should be placed near but not on top of each other
- The two are mixed with the cement spatula using the flat part of the instrument and uniform pressure
- The mixture is consolidated into a mass to check for consistency, which should be creamy for luting applications and similar to putty if needed as an insulating base or intermediate restorative material
- The material is transferred to the dentist under the individual's chin using a plastic filling instrument
- The spatula and plastic filling instrument are both wiped off after use
- If a paper pad was used, the top paper is removed; if a glass slab is used, it is cleaned with alcohol or orange solvent

TWO-PASTE SYSTEM MIXING

The dental assistant mixes, distributes, and either places (if locally allowed) or aids the dentist in placing these preparations.

- Two-paste systems are generally used for temporary bonding
- They consist of an accelerator and a base
- Each paste is spread parallel to the other along a paper pad
- A cement spatula is used to mix the two until the two are of a creamy texture suitable for luting
- This process is very fast (about 15 minutes) as is the setting time (5 minutes or less)
- The material is put in place with the plastic filling instrument
- The cement spatula is wiped off with a gauze sponge

POLYCARBOXYLATE CEMENTS

Polycarboxylate cements are utilized for permanent cementation of orthodontic bands and brackets in addition to other applications. Polycarboxylate cements consist of two portions that are mixed.

- The first is a powder containing primarily zinc oxide with smaller amounts of magnesium oxide and stannous fluoride
- The second is a thick liquid made up of polycyclic acid copolymer in water
- Polycarboxylate cements adhere chemically to the teeth and mechanically to the restoration
- They are relatively strong and non-irritating to the pulp
- The chemical reaction does not release heat
- These cements must be prepared and used quickly as they have a mixing time of a minute or less and an operational time of approximately three minutes
- Unutilized cement should be discarded when it appears dull or sinewy

POLYCARBOXYLATE CEMENTS MIXING

Mixing is done by the dental assistant.

- Powder is placed on one side of a paper pad or glass slab and drops of the liquid on the other
- Manufacturer's directions should indicate the ratio of drops to scoops of powder
- The relative amount of water added is less if a base consistency is desired than if the preparation is to be used for bonding
- The powder is quickly incorporated into the liquid with some pressure for wetting
- The mixture should have a glossy texture
- It should adhere to the spatula somewhat if raised an inch for luting purposes and should be stickier for use as a base
- The mixture should be applied with about 3 minutes before it develops a dull and/or sinewy appearance
- The spatula is wiped off with wet gauze or bathed in 10% NaOH if the cement has dried
- The paper pad is disposed of after use

GLASS IONOMER CEMENTS

There are many types of glass ionomer cements.

- Type I, which has a fine grain and chemically binds to the tooth, is the one used for orthodontic bonding as well as closing up fissures and pits
- Type II is coarser and is utilized for certain kinds of restorations
- Another type is any reinforced admixture containing glass ionomers; it is generally used with silver or amalgam restorations for crown or core buildups
- Unless reinforced, these cements come as a silicate glass powder containing calcium, fluoride, and aluminum, and an aqueous suspension of polycyclic acid
- Glass ionomer cements are quite strong, bond both chemically and mechanically to the teeth, discharge fluoride, and are relatively non-irritating
- While the setting and working times are short, about 1 and 2 minutes respectively, these cements do not set completely for about a day
- Resin-reinforced glass ionomer cements are stronger, less water-soluble, and more adherent

GLASS IONOMER CEMENT MIXING

The dental assistant should rinse and evacuate the patient's mouth first.

- The powder and then the liquid portions are dispensed onto a paper pad or cool glass stab
- It is important to immediately recap the liquid to avoid evaporation
- Working quickly, the assistant moves a portion of the powder into the liquid with a flexible stainless-steel spatula and mixes and incorporates the remaining powder until the proper consistency is achieved
- If the cement is to be used for luting (as for orthodontic work), the texture should be creamy and glossy
- If it is to be used as a base, then the consistency should be stickier
- The mixture is transferred to the dentist under the individual's chin with the plastic filling instrument
- Cleanup involves wiping off the instruments with a moistened gauze and disposal of the top paper
- If glass ionomer capsules are used instead, the seal between the powder and liquid sides is broken in an activator and the tablets are mixed for about 10 seconds on an amalgamator
- The capsule is placed in a dispenser and transferred to the dentist for application
- It is then discarded and the equipment is disinfected

CALCIUM HYDROXIDE CEMENTS

Calcium hydroxide cements are generally just placed in thin layers to protect the pulp by gently chafing the pulp enough to encourage secondary dentin formation.

- They are also used as liners under restorations
- They are not very strong
- The formulations contain other chemicals in addition to the calcium hydroxide and may be either self- or light-curing
- The most common system consists of two pastes, one of which is the base and the other the catalyst for the reaction
- With a two-paste system, equivalent small quantities of base and catalyst are dispensed onto a paper pad
- The two are blended quickly (up to 15 seconds) using a small ball-ended instrument or explorer and a circular motion until a consistent color is achieved
- The implement is transferred on the pad to the dentist under the person's chin
- The duration before setting can be from 2 to 7 minutes, depending on the preparation
- The instrument is wiped off between applications and afterwards and the paper pad is discarded

CAVITY VARNISH

Cavity varnishes are used to close up dentin tubules generally before an amalgam restoration.

- They are applied in a thin layer to the dentin
- All preparations contain some type of resin
- Universal varnishes can be utilized under any restoration materials
- Varnishes that include organic solvents are called copal varnishes and are only appropriate under metal fillings

- Varnishes are one of the weakest types of restorative materials, but they are impenetrable to oral fluids and are useful against microleakage or infiltration of cement acids into the dentin
- Cavity varnishes are prepared and, if allowed by law, applied by the dental assistant
- The patient's mouth should be clean and dry
- Two coats of varnish are generally applied using two small cotton pellets and two cotton pliers
- While holding it in one pair of pliers, the first pellet is moistened with the varnish
- The varnish must be recapped to avoid evaporation
- Extra varnish is dabbed off with gauze, and the desired surface is coated using the cotton pellet
- After drying, the procedure is repeated with the second pellet and pliers
- Pellets are discarded and the pliers are washed with provided solvent

Resin Cement

Resin cements are made up of bisphenol A-glycidyl methacrylate (BIS-GMA) or dimethacrylate resins in combination with low-viscosity monomers and sometimes fluoride.

- The cements do not bond directly to metal or ceramics
- Instead an etchant must first be applied to the tooth surface or a silane coupling agent must be used to achieve mechanical or chemical bonding respectively
- Resin cements are used for a variety of applications
- The curing method is related to the application
- Self- or chemical-cured cements, which have an initiator and activator that are mixed, are used with metal restoration materials or endodontic posts
- Orthodontic brackets and porcelain/resin restorations or veneers indicate use of light cured materials, which are supplied in syringes
- There are also dual-cured materials that come in two parts that are mixed followed by light-curing after application
- There are polyacid-modified compomer cements with similar properties

Etchant and Resin Cement Placement

The tooth surface should be thoroughly cleaned beforehand and the area cleaned and segregated with cotton rolls.

- The dental assistant prepares the etchant applicator and holds it on the tooth surface per manufacturer's specifications, usually up to about 30 seconds
- The etchant could also be transferred to and applied by the dentist. With the dual-curing method of resin cement placement, the tooth is then dried and the adhesive applied
- The resin components, the initiator and activator, are quickly mixed on a paper pad with a stainless-steel spatula to a uniform, creamy consistency
- The assistant transfers the pad near to the patient along with the plastic filling instrument
- The placement is done by the dentist
- The assistant sets up the curing light
- Actual curing or hardening may be done by the dentist or assistant using the curing light and a protective shield or glasses when the light is on
- Gauze sponges are used for cleanup and disposables are thrown out

BONDING AGENTS

Bonding agents are materials that are used for adherence of restoration materials to either dentin or enamel.

- They are also referred to as adhesives or bonding resins
- The main constituents of bonding agents are low-viscosity resins and sometimes fillers, enhancers or fluoride
- Most preparations are light- or dual-cured. In order for bonding to occur, some sort of surface alteration or scoring needs to occur before the bonding agent can penetrate the surface and form a mechanical bond
- For enamel bonding, the first step is acid etching using phosphoric acid
- Bonding to the more-sensitive, organic and water-filled dentin is achieved by initially slashing the dentin with a bur and then using an etchant to eliminate the resulting smear layer

BONDING AGENT PLACEMENT

Bonding systems usually consist of the acid etchant, primer or conditioner, and the adhesive or bonding agent.

- The dental assistant is responsible for preparation and transfer of materials and maintenance of a dry and clean area
- If the procedure is in close contact with the pulp, the first step is placement of lining cement such as calcium hydroxide
- The etchant is then applied to the enamel and then the dentin
- Manufacturer's instructions generally indicate the application time
- The tooth is rinsed
- A brush or disposable applicator is used to apply a primer which moistens the dentin and seeps into the tubules
- The bonding agent is then put on and solidified using a curing light
- Disposable tips or brushes are thrown away

ALGINATE IMPRESSION MATERIAL

Alginate is a general term for irreversible hydrocolloid impression materials.

- These materials are used to make impressions for diagnostic casts and study models
- Their main application in orthodontic work is as negative models for preparation of casts that can be used to formulate orthodontic appliances
- Hydrocolloid impressions are also taken to make opposite models for prosthetics, temporary restorations, bleach trays, custom trays, and mouth guards
- The main ingredient is marine-derived potassium alginate
- It is soluble in water, forming a thick liquid or sol
- When another component, calcium sulfate is added, solidification (a gel) occurs
- Hydrocolloid impression materials also contain trisodium phosphate, which slows down setting time, fillers such as diatomaceous earth or zinc oxide for strength, and potassium titanium fluoride

ADVANTAGES AND DISADVANTAGES

Alginate is extensively used because it is easy, cheap, and comfortable to use.

- It sets quickly, and little equipment is needed
- Its elastic properties make it ideal for making impressions where there are recessed areas
- Both tissue and teeth imprints can be taken
- The major disadvantage is the possibility of some inaccuracy in the impression due to changes in water content
- Heat, dryness, or contact with air can result in syneresis or shrinkage of the material
- Water gain can result in imbibition or an enlargement of the measurements of the impression
- Tissue areas being imprinted may be distorted because of the thickness of the material
- Other impression materials, such as elastomeric ones, are more accurate

PARAMETERS FOR THE STORAGE

Irreversible hydrocolloid impression materials or alginate come packaged in various forms.

- These include hermetic plastic containers with foil or plastic bags inside containing the powder (along with measuring tools for water), mixtures in sealed bags, or similar mixtures used with a dispensing unit
- The materials should be stored in areas where they will not be exposed to moisture or excessive heat
- Shelf life is usually about a year
- The method of mixing the powder and water is usually specified by the manufacturer
- In general, the ratio between the two is 1:1, but two scoops of powder and two portions of water are used for mandibular impressions while three of each is required for maxillary ones
- If too little water is added, the mixture will be too thick
- If too much water is added, the mixture will be too thin

SETTING TIMES

The period between which the water is added to the powder and the total setting of the mixture is the gelatin time.

- This includes approximately one minute of working time for Type II regular-set alginate and less for fast-set Type I
- Setting time is approximately 1-2 minutes or 2 to 4½ minutes for Types I and II respectively if the impression is taken at normal room temperature (about 70°F)
- Both working and setting times are shortened at higher temperatures and lengthened at lower temperatures
- For example, if cool water is used, working and setting times are increased
- In general, Type I is useful for children or people who tend to gag whereas the slower setting Type II is convenient for more difficult insertions or in situations where there is only one operator

BOWLS, SPATULAS, AND TRAYS

Dispensing units using premixed units require only dispensing tips, and the mixture is distributed directly into the tray.

- When mixing of the powder and water is done, special flexible rubber bowls and throwaway spatulas (generally two-sided for mixing of alginate or plaster) are used
- The bowl is sterilized or sanitized afterwards
- There are also disposable spatulas and bowls with markings for water measurement
- There are metal impression trays that must be sterilized after use and disposable plastic trays
- Most have perforations to allow material through and keep it in place
- There are also un-perforated rim lock trays with rims to hold the impression material in place
- Trays come in various sizes and should be selected so that they fit the person's mouth with room for 2 mm of the hydrocolloid
- They should also reach several millimeters posterior to the molar area; if they do not, they can be extended using wax strips (beading)

ALGINATE IMPRESSION PREPARATION

If legally allowed, these procedures are done by the dental assistant.

- The patient should be sitting up
- The patient's mouth is rinsed and evacuated and impression trays are tested for size
- If the selected tray does not extend beyond the molars, wax beading is done at the borders
- The mandibular model should be prepared first
- Two measurements of room temperature water are added to one flexible mixing bowl followed by two scoops of water in another
- Generally, the powder needs to be fluffed beforehand
- The powder is then added to the water and mixed with the spatula first by stirring and then by applying pressure with the smooth side of the spatula on the side of the basin
- Mixing time should be about 30-45 or 60 seconds for fast or regular set preparations respectively
- A creamy, uniform consistency is desired
- The preparation is put in the impression tray starting from the lingual sides
- The flat edge (and sometimes also a moist, gloved hand) is used for consolidation of the material
- Maxillary impressions, which have a greater tendency to cause choking, are prepared similarly later except that 3 measurements of water and 3 scoops of powder are used

IMPRESSION PROCEDURE

In certain states, the dental assistant is legally allowed to take alginate impressions.

- If this is the case, after preparation of the alginate (discussed elsewhere), the operator faces the patient to take the mandibular impression
- First the right cheek is drawn back slightly and unused alginate is spread over the occlusal surfaces
- The impression tray is turned over with the alginate facing the teeth and inserted through the lips one side at a time until it is centered above the teeth
- The back portion of the tray is settled into the teeth first

- At this point, the patient needs to lift and move the tongue to ensure the alveolar process is part of the imprint
- The operator pulls out the person's lip and concludes placing the tray down while pushing toward the back
- The tray is held in place with a finger on each side toward the back and the patient's lip around the tray near the handle
- The alginate is set when it is stiff and fixed
- The maxillary impression tray is loaded similarly except that the tray faces upward and a little of the alginate in the tray needs to be removed from the palate region before insertion

PROCEDURES FOR REMOVAL AND DISINFECTION

Removal is begun by using the fingers of one hand to break the seal between the tissues of the lips and cheek and the tray.

- The other hand is used to shield the opposite arch
- The tray is abruptly removed with a snapping motion either by pulling up or down for the mandibular or maxillary impression
- The tray is turned a bit sideways for removal
- Surplus alginate is removed from the mouth with the evacuator and from the face with a tissue
- The individual should rinse his or her mouth
- The impression should be examined for accuracy and then rinsed with tap water and sprayed with an approved surface disinfectant, such as an iodophor
- Alginate impressions that are not poured into casts immediately (within 20 minutes) should be enclosed in a labeled, covered container until use
- Sometimes the impression is wrapped first in a moist towel, which can lead to water intake and distortion over time

ACCURATE ALGINATE IMPRESSION CHARACTERISTICS

Accurate alginate impressions are centered over the central incisors, include all essential areas, and illustrate well-defined anatomic detail of both teeth and tissues.

- The teeth should not pierce through to the tray, which is caused by pushing the tray up or down too far
- The imprint should not have tears, bubbles, or empty spaces. It should encompass the vestibule regions and have what is known as a good peripheral or marginal roll
- Certain features should be evident
- For the mandibular impression, these are retromolar area, the lingual frenum, and the mylohyoid ridge region
- For the maxillary impression, these are the tuberosities and the palate regions

REVERSIBLE HYDROCOLLOID IMPRESSION MATERIAL

Reversible hydrocolloid impression material, also known as agar-agar, is similar in makeup to alginate.

- The difference is that setting is achieved through a chemical reaction
- The material is transformed from a gel to sol state by boiling for 10 minutes in a hydrocolloid conditioner unit

- It is maintained in a liquid state in a 150°F water bath until about 5 minutes before use at which time it is moved to a 110°F water bath
- Further cooling to convert the material back to a gel is done in the mouth using hoses connected to the dental unit
- Reversible hydrocolloid materials are quite accurate, making them useful for final impressions and other applications requiring detail
- The disadvantages include additional equipment to be bought, longer preparation and setting (10 minutes), and distortion over time if exposed to environmental changes

REQUIRED PACKAGING AND EQUIPMENT

A three-compartment hydrocolloid conditioning unit is used.

- The separate sections all contain clean water maintained at different temperatures
- Looking toward the unit and going from the left, the partitions are the boiling bath (150°F, 66°C), the storage bath (usually 110°F, 45°C), and the conditioning bath (water-cooled tray)
- The impression material is provided in collapsible plastic tubes or syringes, which are shuttled between the three compartments after the appropriate time
- If tubes are used, they are positioned upside down with tips tightly in place into each compartment
- Syringes have special holding cases for the cartridge
- Time must either be set digitally or watched by the dental assistant, particularly the boiling time (10 minutes) and conditioning bath (5 minutes)
- The tray must be cool enough for insertion to avoid burning the patient's mouth. Otherwise, the taking of the impression is fairly similar to the use of alginate except that the setting time is longer, about 10 minutes

ELASTOMERIC IMPRESSION MATERIALS

Elastomeric impression materials are more flexible than other types.

- This means they are less prone to tearing and distortion upon removal
- They are also relatively impervious to temperature changes
- There are three general types of elastomeric impression materials: polysulfide, silicone, and polyether
- Each type is prepared by mixing a catalyst or accelerator and a base material, engendering a process called polymerization
- During the polymerization process, the material converts from a paste into a rubber-like, elastic mass
- Elastomeric impression materials are mixed using either a mixing pad and spatula or an extruder gun to which cartridges of base and catalyst and a mixing tip are attached externally

PROS AND CONS

The pros and cons of blastomeric impression materials are as follows:

- Polysulfide - It comes as a two-paste system, with a base of thiodol polysulfide rubber and filler and a catalyst of lead peroxide. Material is fairly stable after setting, is very precise, and has a long shelf-life. However, it has a sulfurous odor, stains, and a long setting time (at least 10 minutes)

- Silicone - It comes as two color-coded putties, a base of polysiloxane or polyvinyl siloxanes, and a catalyst. The putties are usually mixed and dispensed using an extruder gun. Silicone impression materials are highly accurate, stable, odorless, tasteless, and do not shrink or change measurements. They are relatively expensive
- Polyether - It comes as a color-coded two paste system. The pastes (base and catalyst) are spread in parallel on a paper pad and mixed with a spatula. Polyether systems are quite accurate and stable

POLYSULFIDE IMPRESSION PROCEDURES

Polysulfide impressions are taken by the dentist with one or two assistants supporting.

- The patient is sitting up
- The patient's mouth is rinsed and evacuated
- Two different mixtures are prepared by separate individuals, one for loading onto a syringe and another for loading onto the impression tray
- Parallel, non-touching lines of base and accelerator pastes are dispensed onto two paper pads
- Each is mixed using a spatula with the mixing of the syringe preparation initiated about a minute before that for the tray
- The syringe preparation is put into an impression syringe that has an attached tip (but has had the cylinder removed) by forcing it into the barrel using the working end
- The plunger is inserted and the syringe is transferred to the dentist who applies the material to the prepared tooth
- The tray mixture is loaded into the impression tray with a spatula, smoothed out, and passed to the dentist for insertion
- The tray is held in place for setting a minimum of 6 minutes
- The spatula is cleaned by pulling the material off followed by sterilization
- The paper sheet and disposables are discarded

TWO-STEP SILICONE IMPRESSION PROCEDURES

The dental assistant supports the dentist.

- The patient is sitting up
- Vinyl gloves are suggested
- Silicone impression materials come as two color-coded putties and scoops (base and catalyst) or a putty base plus catalyst in liquid dropper form
- Equivalent amounts are blended and molded into a homogenous patty; this material is mixed and loaded into a stock tray with adhesive within about 30 seconds
- A dent is forged where the affected teeth are to be placed; a plastic spacer sheet is put over the tray, and it is placed in the patient's mouth
- The tray and spacer are removed after about 3 minutes and allowed to set more for a preliminary impression
- A retraction cord is positioned over the desired tooth in preparation for the final impression
- The extruder gun, which mixes and dispenses a lighter body silicone preparation, is used
- A mixing tip is used to force some of the material into the preliminary impression tray, and an intraoral delivery tip is used to injection some around the prepared tooth after retraction cord removal
- The dentist places and holds the tray in place a minimum of 3 minutes until set
- The impression is removed, rinsed, gently died, and disinfected

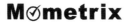

BITE REGISTRATION PROCEDURES

Bite registrations are performed by the dental assistant under supervision or by the dentist aided by the assistant.

- Materials that can be used include bite registration wax or polysiloxane
- The patient is seated upright
- The patient should be taught how to bite in occlusion before the registration
- If bite registration wax is used, the correct length is determined; it is warmed up and softened with water or a torch, and then it is put on the mandibular occlusal edges
- If polysiloxane is utilized, an extruder gun with disposable tip is used force the material right onto the occlusal surfaces
- The assistant watches as the patient bites with proper occlusion as previously directed
- The patient holds the occlusion for a minute or two while the wax cools or until the polysiloxane hardens
- The bite material is taken out, disinfected, labeled, and stored for later use

POLYETHER IMPRESSION PROCEDURES

The two pastes containing the base and catalyst are spread in parallel lines onto a paper pad.

- They are quickly mixed (30 seconds or less) using a spatula, put in the impression tray, and handed to the dentist for the preliminary impression he or she positions the tray and holds it about 3 minutes in the patient's mouth before removal
- About 2 minutes into this process, the tray is moved around
- For the final impression, the base, catalyst, and sometimes a consistency modifier (for thinning) are mixed and forced into the open end of an injection syringe
- This material is put into the preliminary impression, and the tray is reintroduced into the individual's mouth
- It is kept there about 4 minutes and then removed abruptly with a snapping motion, rinsed, dried, and disinfected for 10 minutes with 2% glutaraldehyde
- Sometimes only final polyether impressions are made

Laboratory Materials and Practices

GYPSUM MATERIALS

Gypsum materials are used to make impressions that can be used to make dental models.

- All gypsum products are made from mined hard rock that has been heated to remove water
- This process is known as calcination, which changes the ratio of calcium sulfate to water from 1:2 to 2:1; this represents a change from calcium sulfate dihydrate to hemihydrates
- The resultant material is pulverized and colored; the particle size and color are indicative of the type of gypsum product
- Gypsum materials that have been more extensively ground are denser, stronger, and require less water for wetting and setting
- When water is added to the particles, they convert back to the dihydrate form discharging heat in an exothermic reaction
- Setting is virtually complete when the model is cool to the touch, although complete setting may take a day
- The setting time is reversely related to the water temperature
- The water-to-powder ratio is crucial as it determines strength and fluidity and cannot be changed once setting has begun

GYPSUM PRODUCTS TYPES AND OPTIMAL WATER-TO-POWDER RATIO USE

Gypsum dental products fall primarily into 5 types. Proceeding from Type I to Type VI, the particles are finer, denser, stronger, and require less water for optimal setting. *They are as follows:*

Note that another classification, orthodontic stone, is actually a combination of type II laboratory plaster and type III laboratory stone. Plaster is calcinated by an open kettle technique making the particles very irregular and permeable, whereas die stone is processed by autoclaving with calcium chloride making them denser and more uniform; plaster and stone are known as beta- and alpha-hemihydrate respectively.

Type	Main use	Optimal mL water/100 grams powder
Type I - Impression plaster	impressions	60 mL
Type II - Model or laboratory plaster	casts/models	50 mL
Type III - Laboratory stone	casts/models	30 mL
Type IV - Die stone	strong or dyed models	24 mL
Type V - High-strength, high-expansion die stone	strong or dyed models	18 to 22 mL

PLASTER POURING PROCEDURES

The dental assistant executes these procedures.

- He or she measures out 50 ml of room temperature water into one flexible mixing bowl
- One hundred grams of plaster is weighed into another flexible bowl
- The powder is transferred into the bowl with the water and permitted to dissolve
- This makes a type II model or laboratory plaster
- The particles are blended with a metal spatula for about a minute
- Further mixing is done by pressing and rotating the bowl on a vibrator platform set at low to medium speed
- This process also brings air bubbles that form to the top

- The desired consistency is creamy and smooth, but thick enough to remain in position
- This should be achieved with several minutes on the vibrator

POURING PROCEDURES FOR A STUDY MODEL

This is done by the dental assistant.

- As soon as the plaster has been mixed, it is poured into the alginate impression
- The alginate impression is held over a vibrator on low or medium speed while plaster is added starting at the back of one side of the arch
- The plaster should stream down the back of the impression
- More plaster is added until it flows toward the front teeth to the other arch and out the other end, thus, permeating the anatomical part of the model
- The impression is taken off the vibrator at that point, and the rest of the impression is packed with plaster
- At the end, the impression is briefly vibrated again for amalgamation
- This is the anatomic portion of the model
- If an art portion is to be added, the surface should retain small drops of plaster

ART PORTION POURING PROCEDURES

This is the responsibility of the dental assistant after he or she has poured the anatomical portion of the study model.

- The anatomical portion sets for 5 to 10 minutes
- The flexible rubber or disposable bowl is cleaned and prepared for mixing more plaster
- The ratio of water to powder for the art portion is 40 mL per 100 grams of powder (thicker than the 50 mL/100gm used for the anatomical portion)
- A spatula is used to put the mixture on a glass slab or paper towel creating a base
- The anatomical part of the model is turned over onto the base and positioned such that the tray handle is parallel to the slab or paper
- Surplus plaster is scooped along the edges to fill gaps
- This is the two-pour method
- The art portion can also be poured right after the anatomical part is filled by a single-pour technique
- The model is allowed to set for 40 minutes to an hour; plaster on the outside of the tray is cut off with a laboratory knife, and the model is separated from the impression by holding the tray and lifting upwards

TRIMMING DIAGNOSTIC CASTS OR STUDY MODELS

The dental assistant should wear safety glasses.

- The dry models are wet in flexible mixing bowls
- The assistant should check to see whether the base is parallel to the counter and occlusal plane, and if not, it should be trimmed using the model trimmer
- This is done by using even pressure on the trimming wheel while supporting the hands on the trimmer table
- The maxillary and mandibular models are set together in occlusion to examine further for parallelism
- Once the two are parallel, a pencil line is drawn in back of the retromolar area on the model whose posterior teeth extend back the furthest

- The back of that model is trimmed off at that indicated point perpendicular to the base
- The two models are repositioned in occlusion and held in place while the untrimmed model is cut off at a right angle to its base and at the same spot as the opposing one
- Lines are then drawn to trim off in succession the side areas, anterior cuts, and the heel portion (described elsewhere)
- The following procedure is then followed: the tongue area is trimmed with a laboratory knife; plaster is used to fill in holes; wet sandpaper is used for further smoothing; a model gloss is applied; and the model is polished and labeled

TRIMMING PROCEDURES

For side trimming, lines are marked and cuts made on both models about 5 mm from and parallel to a line between the edge of the model and center of the premolars for the mandible or the cuspids for the maxilla.

- Anterior cuts are then made on the maxillary model along a line from the midline to the area between the canine and cuspid on each quadrant
- The line may have to be protruded outward if teeth are in the way
- For the mandibular model, the anterior cuts back to each cuspid area should be more curved
- Heel cuts are small trimmed edges in the back on either side of each model that extend toward the center of the back

TRIMMED DIAGNOSTIC CAST OR STUDY MODEL CHARACTERISTICS

These casts are usually shown to patients.

- They should be trimmed to certain specifications and look professionally prepared
- Approximately two-thirds of the model should be the anatomical portion and the other third should be the art portion or base for a total depth of 1½ inches (1 and ½ inch respectively)
- Displayed in occlusion, the total height should be 3 inches
- Each model should be symmetrically cut using the angles described elsewhere
- Casts placed in occlusion should be capable of maintaining that relationship when placed on their ends together
- If they fall apart, they are not trimmed properly

ARTICULATOR

Articulators are frames symbolizing the jaws.

- They are attached to study models to keep the models in occlusion and move them
- They are useful for examination of malocclusion
- One of the most common types is the Stephan articulator, which is designed to demonstrate both up-and-down and sideward movements
- It has hinges corresponding to the temporomandibular joints

- A wax bite is placed temporarily to determine correct occlusion
- The base of each model is scored, and then they are connected to bows on the device with additional impression plaster

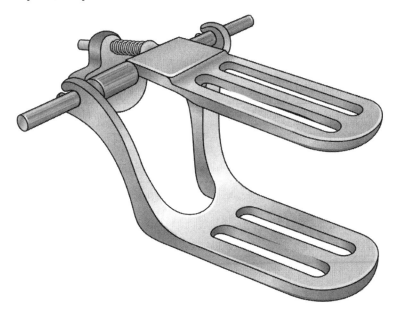

DENTAL WAXES

There are three general categories of dental waxes.

- The first, pattern wax, is represented by two relatively hard waxes, inlay and baseplate waxes
- Inlay wax comes in dark sticks that are melted and placed on a die to create a pattern for a restoration or heated to vaporization with the lost wax technique
- Baseplate wax comes in sheets that are heated for use as denture bases
- The next category is temporary processing waxes
- These include the following: soft boxing wax, used to enclose impressions to keep gypsum in place; sticky wax, which sticks to many types of surfaces when melted for temporary repair jobs; and utility wax, which has adhesive and malleable properties at room temperature, making it ideal for relieving patient discomfort (e.g., over orthodontic brackets)
- The last major category is impression or bite registration waxes, which usually incorporate copper or aluminum particles
- Other waxes include hard blocks of study wax that can be whittled and undercut wax which is placed in undercuts before making impressions

CUSTOM TRAY MATERIAL

Custom trays are generally made from some type of acrylic or other resin or a thermoplastic substance. The 4 main types of materials are as follows:

- Self-curing acrylic tray resin - This system combines a polymer powder with a liquid catalyst or monomer initiating a process called polymerization and exothermic release of heat. Complete setting to a very hard state takes about a day
- Light-cured acrylic tray resin - Material is similar to above but remains malleable until a special curing light is activated, which initiates the polymerization and setting much faster

- Vacuum-formed custom trays - These use heavy, stiff sheets of plastic resin. The resin is hung within a special unit and heated until soft. The sheet is then released onto the model as vacuum pressure is applied
- Thermoplastic materials - Beads or buttons are softened and made pliant through exposure to heat, usually warm water. After shaping, hardening occurs as heat disperses

CUSTOM TRAY CRITERIA

A custom tray is usually fabricated in order to make an accurate impression.

- Therefore, the tray must be durable enough to hold the material during positioning and removal
- It should be smoothed and shaped to the individual's arch
- Ideally, it should allow the impression material to fill with consistent thickness in all regions of the arch
- The tray should be adaptable to any type of dentition from an edentulous condition to full dentition as well as any other type of unusual area
- Trays that have stops in the spacer to grip the impression material in certain areas are a good design and provide greater accuracy for the impression

OUTLINING THE MARGINS AND PREPARING THE CAST

This is the first step in constructing a custom tray.

- It is done by the dental assistant on a working plaster or stone cast
- Generally, a blue line is drawn in the deepest area of the entire margin and a red line for wax spacer placement is drawn 1 to 2 mm above that
- This corresponds to about 2 to 3 mm below the tooth margin or above the lowest point of the vestibule if edentulous
- Spacers are made of pink baseplate wax, a special molding material, or wet paper towels
- Any recessed undercuts in the model are plugged
- The spacer material is heated, shaped to the red line, and trimmed to the line with a laboratory knife
- Stops or holes are cut at intervals on the top edges of the spacer to permit the passage of impression material
- The top of the spacer is draped with aluminum foil if self-cured resin is being used to dissipate heat and facilitate removal of wax at the end
- Sometimes a separating material is painted over the spacer

RESIN MIXING AND CONTOURING A SELF-CURED ACRYLIC RESIN CUSTOM TRAY

Outlining of the margins and preparation of the cast are described elsewhere.

- The dental assistant then mixes the self-curing resin components, the powder polymer, and the liquid catalyst in a wax-lined paper cup with a wooden tongue blade until the mixture is uniform
- The measuring tools and proportions for mixing should be specified by the manufacturer
- The initial set or polymerization takes about 2 to 3 minutes
- Petroleum jelly is applied to the palms and the cast
- The dental assistant takes the malleable resin and hand manipulates it into a doughy patty or roll for a maxillary or mandibular arch

- A little is reserved to make a handle later. The resin patty or roll is inserted over and extended slightly beyond (1 to 2 mm) the wax spacer
- For the maxillary tray, this means inclusion of the palatal area
- It is manually contoured with a rolled edge; use of the laboratory knife is permitted but less desirable
- The handle material is molded and attached to the front of the tray near the midline using a drop of the monomer catalyst liquid

FINISHING PROCEDURES OF A SELF-CURED ACRYLIC RESIN CUSTOM TRAY:

- The custom tray is removed after 8 to 10 minutes of setting from the model and wax spacer
- The wax is cleaned out by melting or using a spatula, hot water, and a toothbrush
- The outside edges of the tray are trimmed later using an acrylic bur
- Safety glasses should be worn
- This should not be done until the material is completely set, which takes at least a half hour
- The tray is cleaned, disinfected, and labeled
- Before the impression is taken, two thin coats of impression adhesive are painted onto the inside of the tray and along the margins
- Sometimes holes are made in the tray using a round bur to further secure the impression material into it

VACUUM-FORMED ACRYLIC RESIN CUSTOM TRAY

The dental assistant prepares the previously-made cast by immersing it in warm water for up to a half hour.

- This gets rid of surface air bubbles
- Spacers are added if specified, and the outer margin is outlined
- A special vacuum-forming unit is used with a platform on which the prepared cast is placed
- The unit also has 2 frames that special acrylic resin sheets are secured between
- These hang above the platform
- One of the frames contains a heating element
- It is turned on causing the resin sheet to droop downward
- When the resin hangs down about an inch, the operator pulls the frames down over the cast using the handles on the sides
- The vacuum is activated right after the resin drops over the cast; the heat is turned off, and the vacuum is kept on for a minute or two
- Once the tray cools, it is taken off the frame, released from the model, and trimmed to the preferred form with a laboratory scissors
- A handle is cut and attached using a torch
- The tray is cleaned, disinfected and labeled

PROSTHODONTICS

Prosthodontics or prostheses are artificial parts created in the dental laboratory to replace missing teeth or tissues.

- They can be fixed or removable
- Fixed prostheses are designed to integrate into the natural dentition and are maintained through regular brushing and flossing

- The purposes they serve include restoration of chewing ability, prevention of teeth movement by providing underlying support, speech improvement, and promotion of oral hygiene
- Fixed prostheses may be used for other esthetic reasons
- Crowns, inlays, outlays, bridges, and veneers are examples of fixed prosthodontics
- Removable prosthodontics fit into two categories:
  - partial dentures replacing one or more teeth in an arch
  - complete or full dentures that take the place of all teeth in one arch
- Partial dentures are held in place by underlying tissues and other teeth while full dentures are supported by gingival and oral mucosal tissues, alveolar ridges, and the hard palate

DENTAL PROSTHESES

Fixed prostheses are maintained by brushing and flossing.

- Toothbrushes selected should be soft, multi-tufted, and small enough to access all areas
- Bridges can be cleaned by using a bridge threader to insert dental floss underneath
- Interproximal brushes and tips are also available
- Dental implants, which are titanium devices or screws that fuse with bone tissue by bonding (osseointegration), should be brushed with a similar type of brush and a specialized type of floss that is wider and designed to be wrapped around the implant (such as Proxi-Floss)
- Other maintenance measures include use of a plastic interproximal brush, water irrigators for plaque and debris removal, antimicrobial rinses, and a variety of plastic cleaning instruments
- Removable prostheses or dentures should be cleaned with a special denture toothbrush and mild soap or toothpaste
- Tissue under the denture should also be brushed
- Dentures are also taken out and put in cleaning agents to get rid them of stains
- Orthodontic devices should be maintained with specially designed toothbrushes, water irrigation, and often an interproximal brush

ORTHODONTIC BANDS, BRACKETS, OR ARCH WIRES REPAIR

Loose bands are usually visible to the eye or can be felt by the patient.

- The bands slide up and down when probed with a scaler or explorer
- Usually they are just cleansed and recemented
- Sometimes they are repaired by welding with a variation of a soldering iron or other welding equipment
- If bonded brackets work loose from the tooth surface or the pad, they are generally replaced
- Bent or broken arch wires require immediate attention
- Bent wires should be reformed and broken ones should be replaced by the orthodontist

Prevention and Management of Emergencies

DENTAL OFFICE EMERGENCY KIT

Each treatment room should have oxygen inhalation equipment as a self-contained unit (with a green oxygen tank) or through a wall-piped system in association with nitrous oxide gas administration.

- The oxygen tank(s) should be tested weekly
- The dental office emergency kit should contain various devices (in good working order) useful in emergency situations, such as oral airway apparatuses, tracheotomy needles, barriers used with cardiopulmonary resuscitation, tourniquets, and hygienic syringes
- The kit should include various classes of drugs
- Antihistamines are important to counteract allergic reactions; various pill and injectable (like an epi-pen) forms are suggested
- The kit should contain vasodilators such as nitroglycerin to increase blood flow and treat high blood pressure (hypertension), a vasopressor such as Wyamine to treat low blood pressure (hypotension), anti-convulsants such as Diazepam, drugs that block the vagal nerve and increase the pulse rate such as atropine, and analgesic pain relievers
- The medications should be checked for expiration dates periodically and replaced if needed

OXYGEN ADMINISTRATION

The dental assistant can administer oxygen in emergency situations.

- A mobile cart with a unit containing a green oxygen tank is used
- The patient should be in the Trendelenburg position, which is lying on the back with feet raised above chest level
- The oxygen mask is positioned over the person's nose with tubing to the side
- The mask must be fastened firmly
- Oxygen is administered without delay, at a rate of between 2 and 4 liters a minute
- The professional should explain to the patient the proper breathing during the procedure, which is nose breathing with the mouth closed
- During the administration, the assistant should try to calm down and comfort the individual

ADULT RESCUE BREATHING

Rescue breathing in emergency situations may be done by the dental assistant or dentist with assistance.

- Emergency services should also be called before beginning if the patient is orally unresponsive
- Gloves are suggested but not required
- If the person does not appear to be breathing, his or her head should be tilted back, the chin raised, and a resuscitation mouthpiece put in the mouth
- The professional then pinches the nose closed and provides two breaths
- The breaths should make the patient's chest rise
- The person performing the procedure should then listen and observe the chest for breathing
- The pulse should be checked at the closest carotid artery using the middle and forefingers for palpation
- Rescue breathing is done as long as there is a pulse

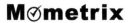

- This is defined as one slow breath every five seconds for a minute followed by checking of the pulse and breathing and repeating the sequence until breathing is re-established or someone else takes over
- Cardiopulmonary resuscitation is indicated if the pulse stops
- The mouthpiece should be thrown out into a biohazard container and the incident documented

CPR ABC's

Cardiopulmonary resuscitation (CPR) is an emergency technique use to revive a person whose heart has stopped beating.

- The process of CPR can be said to follow an ABC (and often D) pattern
- The "A" represents the airway, which must first be opened up to allow air flow
- The "B" signifies breathing, which the rescuer must monitor and work to establish if the patient is not breathing
- The "C" stands for circulation, which the rescuer must check for using the carotid pulse; if there is no pulse, then chest compressions interspersed with slow breaths are used to establish a pulse
- The "D" refers to an adjunct technology called defibrillation, which involves use of an automated external defibrillation (AED) unit if available
- Dental assistants are required to be certified in CPR every two years at the Healthcare Provider Level by either the American Red Cross or the American Heart Association

CPR FOR AN ADULT USING A SINGLE RESCUER

CPR in emergency situations is done by the dental assistant or dentist with assistance.

- Emergency services should also be called before beginning if the patient is orally unresponsive
- Gloves are suggested
- Ideally the patient should be supine or the dental chair can be adapted
- The rescuer first observes, listens, and feels the person for evidence of breathing
- If there is none, the rescuer opens the patient's airway by inclining the head back and raising the chin
- A resuscitation mouthpiece is put in the individual's mouth and the nose is pinched closed
- The rescuer applies two breaths, observes the chest rise, and then tests the pulse for about 15 seconds, using the carotid artery
- If no pulse is present, 4 cycles of chest compression followed by two slow breaths are done
- The chest compressions are performed kneeling at the side using one hand on top of the other and compressing down on the breastbone 15 times quickly
- After each set of 4 cycles, the carotid pulse is tested again
- The 4 cycle sets of compression/breaths followed by checking of the pulse are continued until revival or rescuer substitution
- The mouthpiece is discarded and the procedures documented

AED Unit for Cardiac Arrest

An AED or automated external defibrillation unit is used to revive a person in cardiac arrest.

- Cardiopulmonary resuscitation should be carried out until the unit is ready
- The "analyze" button is pressed first and a sequence of steps must ensue before the unit can be used
- The electrodes of the AED are then connected to the patient as illustrated on the unit
- The rescuer announces that everyone must stay clear of the patient while he or she determines whether an electric shocking is indicated; this is done by pushing the analysis button to get a readout
- CPR should be reestablished if shocking is contraindicated. Otherwise, the unit will have an audible or light means of indicating that is ready to shock the patient
- The AED shows when shocking is occurring
- The pulse should be tested after the third shock
- If there is a pulse, the airway, breathing, and vital signs should be checked
- If not, additional CPR should be done for a minute before rechecking the pulse
- If there is still no pulse, defibrillation is repeated using the analysis button again up to 3 times or 9 more shocks with interspersed checking and CPR (as above)
- The unit will show when shocking is no longer indicated

Foreign Body Airway Obstruction

Since a dental patient is typically lying back with objects slippery from saliva or blood in his or her mouth, there are many opportunities for foreign body airway obstruction (FBAO) to occur.

- The universal distress signal for FBAO is clutching of the throat with both hands and chocking
- If the patient does this, the dentist or assistant should suspend the treatment
- The patient should be persuaded to sit up and cough, but if the patient cannot force out the foreign body, the rescuer should begin the Heimlich maneuver to open the blocked airway
- The Heimlich maneuver is a series of subdiaphragmatic thrusts performed on a standing individual who is conscious
- The rescuer stands behind the patient and wraps his or her arms around the abdomen
- One hand should be made into a fist which is positioned with the thumb side against the center of the patient's abdomen; the other hand is firmly grasped over it
- Swift, upward thrusts are applied until the airway is cleared or the person becomes unconscious

Abdominal Thrusts in an Unconscious Patient

If a patient with foreign body airway obstruction (FBAO) is or becomes unconscious during the Heimlich maneuver, the treatment changes.

- Emergency medical services (EMS) should be contacted without delay
- The individual should be placed on his or her back
- Using gloves, the rescuer should lift the tongue and jaw and then use a finger to go through the mouth and remove the foreign body
- The airway is opened (tilting the head, lifting the chin, pinching the nose), a resuscitation device is inserted into the mouth, and two slow breaths are given
- Repositioning of the head may be required

- If the airway appears to remain obstructed, then abdominal thrusts for expulsion are indicated
- The rescuer straddles the patient's thighs, positions the heels of both hands just below the xiphoid notch at the base of the sternum, and applies up to 5 abdominal thrusts pressing toward the diaphragm
- One hand can be placed on top of the other
- The series of thrusts is continued until the airway is unblocked or EMS arrives to take over

SYNCOPE

Syncope or fainting is basically a loss of consciousness due to decreased blood flow to the brain.

- Syncope is usually caused by stress, which triggers blood flow to the extremities at the expense of flow to the brain
- The individual feels dizzy or nauseated initially
- Lowering the head will increase the blood flow to the brain
- If the patient becomes unconscious but is breathing normally, transferring the patient to the Trendelenburg position (lying back with slightly elevated feet) is useful because blood can stream back to the brain
- If the patient is not breathing naturally, the airway should be opened by inclining the head and raising the chin
- Restrictive clothing or jewelry at the neck should be slackened or removed
- Oxygen is dispensed using an oxygen tank, mask and tubing as a precaution
- If breathing does not resume within 15 seconds, the oxygen mask is taken off and spirits of ammonia are tried
- A vial of ammonia is broken and applied to a gauze sponge, and the sponge is passed under the person's nose for a second or two
- This should stimulate the person to take in air and oxygen and should revive him or her within a minute
- Otherwise, CPR should be started and emergency help called

ASTHMA

Asthma is a respiratory disease.

- It is often due to allergies and is characterized by breathlessness and wheezing upon expiration
- Asthma attacks are most likely to occur in the morning
- A patient with asthma has narrowing in the bronchioles (small airways) in the lung
- During exhalation, the lung collapses and bronchiole narrowing is exacerbated further, making it increasingly difficult to breathe
- The usual treatment is administration of antihistamines such as albuterol using an inhaler
- The individual exhales first and then inhales the bronchodilator drug through the device's mouthpiece while depressing the canister portion
- Bronchodilators expand the bronchioles to enhance air flow
- Usually two inhalations of bronchodilator will allay an attack and improve breathing in about 15 minutes
- Otherwise oxygen should be dispensed and emergency services summoned

ALLERGIC REACTION

An allergic reaction is a response to exposure to some type of foreign agent or antigen.

- When an individual is exposed initially to a foreign antigen, the body's immune system develops antibodies to the antigen
- Subsequent antigenic exposures set off an allergic or hypersensitivity response in which large amounts of histamine and other chemicals are released
- Asthma, discussed on another card, is usually due to an allergic response in the airways
- Anaphylactic shock is another possible manifestation
- Allergens in the bloodstream stimulate histamine release causing an immediate depression in blood pressure, airway constriction, swelling of the throat and tongue, and stomach pain
- Epinephrine must be given right away usually with an epi-pen
- Allergic response can also manifest as skin reactions like edema, erythema, or urticaria, which indicate irritant removal and usually dispensation of antihistamine drugs

HYPERVENTILATION

Hyperventilation is deep and rapid breathing.

- It usually occurs as a result of anxiety
- If a person hyperventilates for any prolonged period of time, he or she becomes faint, develops a loose feeling in the extremities, and cannot take complete breaths
- The person experiences alkalosis or high blood pH, which further exacerbates the anxiety and rapid breathing
- Hyperventilation in a dental patient should be addressed by terminating the procedure, getting the patient to sit up, and allaying the patient's anxieties
- The patient should be instructed to hold his or her breath a few seconds before exhalation, which reverses the alkalosis by getting more carbon dioxide and less oxygen into the blood
- An alternative tactic is having the patient breathe into a paper sack or his or her hands
- The converse is shallow breathing or hypoventilation which can result in CO_2 accumulation in the blood and the need for oxygen

EPILEPTIC ATTACK

Epilepsy is a disorder of the brain in which electrical impulses are disorganized.

- Origins for epilepsy range from head injuries to metabolic imbalances to drug withdrawal
- A person experiencing an epileptic attack has some level of seizure or convulsion
- There are tonic-clonic (grand mal), absence (petit mal), and partial seizures
- The tonic-clonic type, the most common, is characterized by body jerking, twitching, and unconsciousness for about 2 to 5 minutes, usually followed by incontinence and exhaustion; a continuous convulsant seizure is called status epilepticus (EMS should be called)
- An absence seizure is characterized by a brief loss of consciousness and blank staring
- During partial seizures, an epileptic either retains or loses consciousness, referred to as simple or complex
- Both forms manifest primarily as involuntary twitching; the main difference is recall ability
- Absence and partial seizure do not require treatment
- Dental procedures should be stopped and everything should be taken out of the oral cavity during seizures
- Afterwards the patient should lie on the right side with the airway open

Type I and Type II Diabetes Mellitus

Type I or juvenile diabetes mellitus is a hereditary condition in which cells in the pancreas cannot produce insulin.

- Insulin is a hormone that regulates glucose levels in the blood
- Type I diabetics are insulin-dependent, meaning they must receive frequent injections of insulin to avoid a loss of consciousness
- Type II diabetes mellitus patients have a decreased sensitivity to insulin, which also disturbs the blood glucose balance
- Type II diabetes is not considered hereditary and tends to occur later in life
- When too much glucose accumulates in the blood, hyperglycemia occurs
- Hyperglycemia can precipitate attacks of either type with similar symptoms, although type II ones are less severe
- These symptoms include thirst, frequent urination, confusion, nausea, vomiting, and abdominal aches
- Dental procedures should be suspended
- Treatment for Type I diabetics is administration of insulin via insulin pen or portable pump to prevent diabetic acidosis and possible coma
- Type II diabetics usually can control their disease with diet or through the use of oral hypoglycemics

Hypoglycemia

Hypoglycemia is too low a concentration of blood glucose.

- It is generally caused by not eating, overexertion, or stress
- Its symptoms are nervousness, shaking, weakness, cold sweats, and/or hunger
- The treatment goal is to increase the blood sugar level
- When an episode of hypoglycemia occurs in the dental office, treatment should be discontinued and orange juice or another source of sugar should be consumed
- If the person loses consciousness, medical assistance should be called and sugar supplied either by giving a shot of glucagon or applying a sugar source to the buccal mucosa
- Excess amounts of insulin can produce severe hypoglycemia and a critical drop in blood sugar called insulin shock; in this case intravenous glucose is indicated

Angina Pectoris

Angina pectoris and myocardial infarction are two types of cardiovascular emergencies that can result from arteriosclerosis or atherosclerosis.

- Arteriosclerosis is the loss of elasticity in the arteries
- Arteriosclerosis is plaque buildup within the arteries and subsequent narrowing of the arteries, resulting in decreased blood flow
- Angina pectoris is pain in the chest area or base of the neck usually accompanied by increased blood pressure and pulse rate
- The treatment is sublingual administration of nitroglycerin pills or use of nitroglycerin spray to open up the coronary arties and supply the heart with more oxygenated blood
- If an episode of angina pectoris occurs in the dental office, the procedure should be stopped and the patient is usually given oxygen and allowed to take his or her nitroglycerin
- Up to three doses of nitroglycerin spaced at 3 to 5 minute intervals can be taken before diagnosing a myocardial infarction (discussed elsewhere)

MYOCARDIAL INFARCTION

A myocardial infarction (MI) or heart attack is an event in which a portion of heart tissue dies rapidly due to severe blockage or narrowing of the coronary arteries.

- The possible symptoms of MI are angina pectoris, an ashen color, and/or copious sweating
- Chest pain due a myocardial infarction cannot be assuaged with nitroglycerin administration as it can with angina pectoris alone
- If an MI occurs in the dental office, procedures should be terminated and the patient should be repositioned with the head slightly up
- Professionals should work to alleviate the patient's stress
- It is important to contact medical emergency services immediately for transport and administer oxygen and nitroglycerin in the interim
- MI, which is more prevalent in males, smokers, older individuals, and diabetics, can be controlled somewhat through diet, exercise, and lowering stress and blood pressure

CONGESTIVE HEART FAILURE

Congestive heart failure is a condition in which there is a suboptimal ability to pump blood, which causes congestion or fluid retention in the veins.

- The heart cannot supply sufficient oxygenated blood to meet the body's needs
- Congestive heart failure can adversely affect many of the body's systems
- The individual has swollen ankles and legs and trouble breathing
- These patients need to have their head and heart elevated to avoid fluids from being pulled toward them
- They also usually need frequent bathroom breaks because the customary medical treatment for people with congestive heart failure is use of diuretic drugs
- Diuretic drugs enhance urine output and decrease fluid buildup and swelling

STROKE

A stroke is an abrupt cerebrovascular accident.

- There are several types of strokes, all characterized by a sudden stoppage of blood flow to the brain
- Strokes occur because a blood clot causes blockage (known as a cerebral embolism) or a blood vessel in the brain bursts (known as a cerebral hemorrhage)
- Vessel tissues in the brain die and cause a cerebral infarction
- Possible symptoms during a stroke include severe headache, speech loss, dizziness, weakness or paralysis on one side of the body (hemiplegia), and/or loss of consciousness
- If a patient experiences a stroke in the dental office, procedures should be terminated
- Everything should be removed from the patient's mouth, and the person should be repositioned with the head slightly raised
- The EMS should be called while oxygen is given and vital signs are checked until they arrive
- Cardiopulmonary resuscitation may also be necessary

ABSCESSED OR AVULSED TEETH

Abscesses are pus-filled cavities resulting from bacterial infection and inflammation.

- Abscessed or infected teeth are painful due to pressure and edema
- If they are ignored, the infection spreads into the surrounding tissues producing a fistula or passageway leading to the oral cavity
- This fistula alleviates some of the pressure
- Root canal therapy, removal of necrotic pulp, creation of an opening into the pulp chamber, and treatment of the infection are strategies for dealing with abscessed teeth
- Avulsed or forcibly loosened teeth should initially be wrapped in wet gauze and inserted between the teeth and lip or put in milk and then taken to the dental office at once
- The dentist then reattaches the tooth in the socket using adjacent teeth to shore it up
- Primary avulsed teeth are not reattached, however, as infection or ankylosis (fusion of bone and cementum) can result
- Primary teeth that have been displaced to the side or are loose should be repositioned and secured with a temporary splint as soon as possible

FRACTURED TEETH

Broken teeth are addressed according to the amount and type of breakage, the degree of discomfort, and age

- In children, pulp treatment is usually done and a temporary restoration installed before further assessment several months later
- Tooth fractures involving the enamel alone are addressed by smoothing the rough edges
- If the fracture involves both enamel and dentin, then the exposed dentin is covered with glass ionomer, calcium hydroxide, and a bonding agent and composite restoration is done
- If the break is down into the pulp as well, pulp capping or removal is indicated
- If the crown is cracked with exposure of pulp, the suggested treatment, if necessary, is a root canal supplemented by posts and casts in the crown for stabilization and protection

SOFT TISSUE INJURIES

Soft tissue injuries to the oral-facial area can occur easily during dental procedures because the oral cavity is damp and slippery, the patient may shift, or equipment can be dislodged.

- Soft tissue injuries to the area can also be caused outside the office by any contact with a sharp or dull object, electrical burns, or sports injuries
- A situation unique to children is traumatic intrusion or the forcing of freshly erupted teeth back into their sockets after a tumble
- Traumatic intrusion is treated by either permitting the teeth to re-erupt or by moving them and using a splint across adjacent teeth for support
- If traumatic intrusion occurs to primary teeth, the extent of damage to emergent permanent teeth underneath cannot be fully ascertained until they erupt

ALVEOLITIS

When a tooth has been extracted, normally a blood clot forms over the socket.

- Alveolitis or a dry socket occurs when there is no blood clot formation or the clot is rinsed out of the socket exposing nerve endings and making the area susceptible to infection

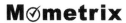

- The therapy for alveolitis is cleansing with saline and stuffing the socket with a gauze strip or sponge drenched in the antiseptic iodoform to relieve pain
- Analgesics may be used as well for palliation
- Medicated dressings are usually replaced in a day or two
- In a surgical setting after extraction, anesthesia may be administered prior to treatment

Loose Permanent or Temporary Crowns

In addition to anatomical and clinical definitions of crown, the term also refers to prostheses that cover the coronal surface of a tooth with broad decay or other problems.

- There are full-cast crowns that enclose the complete coronal surface and partial crowns that cover up to three surfaces of a tooth
- They are usually made of porcelain, gold, stainless steel, or some combination of porcelain and metal
- Loss of a permanent or temporary crown is a dental emergency
- A temporary fix is to use petroleum jelly or orthodontic wax to keep the crown in position
- The individual must be careful during meals not to dislodge the crown
- As soon as possible, the crown should be recemented in place with the appropriate type of cement

Emergency Preparedness Procedures

The role of each person in the dental office during an emergency should be clearly identified.

- For example, the front desk personnel should call for emergency help; the assistant or hygienist should be responsible for getting the oxygen and emergency kit and providing or assisting the dentist with provision of life support activities
- Cross training in various roles should be done, and routine practice drills should be conducted
- Emergency telephone numbers should be clearly posted, including the emergency medical service (EMS) and area fire and police numbers
- A general emergency number is usually 911
- The numbers for nearby doctors, hospitals, and oral surgeons should also be clearly displayed

Topical or Local Anesthetic Complications

Topical anesthetics can cause allergic and toxic reactions.

- Swelling, erythema, ulcerations, and difficulty swallowing or breathing up to a day or more after application indicate an allergic reaction, which should be treated with antihistamines
- Toxic reactions are central nervous system (CNS) complications that occur due to an overdose of topical anesthetic
- The patient initially becomes talkative and anxious, and his or her blood pressure and pulse rates go up; however, the CNS reactions later reverse
- Excessive administration of local anesthetic drugs can also produce similar toxic reactions as well as paresthesia or numbness
- Paresthesia should be documented because it involves nerve damage that can eventually become permanent

DRUG DISTINCTION

Drugs are substances that can alter bodily processes.

- They are used to treat diseases or alleviate pain
- They may be naturally-occurring or created artificially
- Laws require certain drugs to be dispensed only by prescription while others can be obtained over-the-counter (OTC)
- The only professionals licensed to write prescriptions for controlled substances are doctors, dentists, and physician assistants
- While most drugs have potential beneficial effects, they generally also have possible side effects and drug interactions
- Side effects are inadvertent consequences of use of a particular drug
- For example, immunosuppressant drugs used to thwart organ graft rejection also make an individual more susceptible to infection
- Drug interactions are unintentional consequences of the simultaneous use of two or more drugs
- The combination of drugs acts synergistically to magnify, diminish, or change the effects of each
- Drug addiction generally refers to physical dependency on a drug with withdrawal symptoms occurring if it is discontinued

CURRENT DRUG LAWS

Early drug-related laws in the United States were the 1906 Pure Food and Drug Act and later, in 1938, the Pure Food, Drug, and Cosmetic Act, which gave rise to the Food and Drug Administration (FDA). The current applicable drug law in the United States is the Comprehensive Drug Abuse Prevention and Control Act of 1970, which divides drugs into 5 categories or schedules based on their potential for abuse. Briefly the drug schedule is as follows:

- Schedule I drugs - great potential for abuse and no established medical benefit, such as heroin
- Schedule II drugs - great possibility of abuse and dependence but with some known medical benefit; comprised of narcotics (e.g., morphine) and barbiturate (e.g., amphetamines)
- Schedule III drugs - less potential for abuse and having established medical utility; includes other barbiturates, stimulants, depressants, and combinations, including many drugs used in dental practice
- Schedule IV drugs - even less potential for abuse with established medical utility and little possibility of addiction; includes sedatives, anti-anxiety drugs and certain depressants
- Schedule V drugs - slightest potential for abuse, generally dispensed over-the-counter

DRUG ADMINISTRATION

Most drugs or medications are taken via the oral route in the form of pills taken with water or liquids.

- In the dental office, topical administration is common particularly for anesthesia; some sort of ointment or cream is put on the skin or oral mucosa
- Another common route in dentistry is through inhalation of a gas, in particular, nitrous oxide
- Intravenous injection of a drug directly into the vein is a rapid method of getting it into the bloodstream and eliciting a response

- Drugs are sometimes injected intramuscularly, subcutaneously, or intradermally (into muscle tissue, underneath the skin, or below the upper epidermal layer of skin, respectively)
- Sublingual dispensation under the tongue is uncommon in the dental office, but it may apply with nitroglycerin administration for patients having an attack of angina pectoris
- Nitroglycerin may be taken by another route of administration, the transdermal skin patch, which releases medication at a steady rate
- The final route, rectal administration, uses suppositories or enemas and is generally not applicable

TOBACCO, CAFFEINE, OR ALCOHOL

While readily available and legal, all of these substances can be considered drugs, and they all can be addictive.

- People who smoke or chew tobacco expose themselves to the stimulant nicotine
- Nicotine use predisposes individuals to lung and other cancers, including oral cancer
- It also contributes to heart disease and a variety of oral problems, such as tooth staining, periodontal disease, and bad breath
- Usually drinking beverages with caffeine, such as coffee or tea, is safe, but excessive amounts can lead to overstimulation of the heart and nervous system, stomach ulcers, and stained teeth
- Alcoholic beverages contain ethyl alcohol, a known depressant
- If consumed in excessive quantities, alcohol can slow down responses and lead to loss of judgment, coordination and speech
- Alcohol use can lead to dependency, convulsions, delusional behavior, and cirrhosis of the liver

MARIJUANA AND COCAINE

Two widespread illegal drugs are marijuana and cocaine.

- Patients who have taken marijuana recently may have an extremely high heart rate
- The main active ingredient is tetrahydrocannabinol or THC, but the combination of drugs in marijuana makes it equally a stimulant and depressant
- Habitual use can lead to lung tissue damage, reproductive system abnormalities, speech and coordination problems, and lack of motivation
- Currently there is no evidence for physical dependence on marijuana, but people can become emotionally dependent on it
- It is used to reduce nausea in cancer patients and to treat glaucoma
- Cocaine, on the other hand, is addictive both physically and psychologically and is often used in conjunction with other addictive drugs, potentiating its effects and the possibility of drug interactions. It is a stimulant.
- Cocaine use can lead to cardiovascular issues, extreme anxiety, violent conduct, various mental illnesses, and even death

NARCOTIC DRUGS

All narcotic drugs are depressants that have the potential for physical and psychological addiction.

- Two of these narcotic drugs, morphine and codeine, are often administered as analgesics or pain killers
- Morphine is generally used for more severe pain and may be administered intravenously, intramuscularly, or orally
- Occasional use can cause constipation, nausea, and disorientation, but habitual use leads to addiction
- Codeine is used for mild to moderate pain, usually in formulations with other medications
- Its main side effects are tiredness and constipation
- Heroin has no accepted medical use. It is taken intravenously, subcutaneously, or via inhalation
- Individuals who habitually use heroin become addicted and tolerant to it
- Warning signs of heroin use are depressed respiratory and heart rates, constipation, and loss of appetite
- A heroin overdose is an emergency situation characterized by vomiting, diarrhea, shock, and potentially loss of consciousness
- Overdosed heroin addicts should be transferred right away to a hospital where they can be given a narcotic antagonist

HALLUCINOGENS

Hallucinogenic drugs are considered drugs of abuse.

- They cause a person to hallucinate or imagine that he or she is experiencing things that are not really occurring
- Subsequently, the individual has modified brain activity, causing unpredictable or violent behavior
- LSD or lysergic acid diethylamide and its close relative psilocybin are both hallucinogens
- LSD is derived from the fungus ergot and psilocybin comes from mushrooms
- Phencyclidine or PCP is another hallucinogen that has both stimulatory and depressive effects, such as violent conduct, convulsions, nausea, suppression of respiration, and prolonged memory loss
- Mescaline, which is derived from the peyote cactus, does not promote as extreme behavior, but it can cause permanent psychosis

AMPHETAMINE OR BARBITURATE USE

Amphetamines and barbiturates have sort of opposite effects, but both can be addictive.

- Amphetamines are stimulants, increasing heart rate, respiratory rate, and blood pressure
- Aggressive behavior and poor judgment are warnings signs of amphetamine use
- Amphetamines do have an accepted medical use in the treatment of narcolepsy or attention deficit hyperactivity disorder
- Barbiturates slow down brain activity and have a calming or tranquilizing effect
- One barbiturate, phenobarbital, is commonly administered for insomnia, epilepsy, and anxiety (including in the dental office)
- The main issues with barbiturates are dependency and tolerance with long-term use, withdrawal symptoms if taken away after prolonged use, and potentially critical overdosing
- Overdosing can cause disorientation, coma, and death

ANTIBIOTICS SIDE EFFECTS

Antibiotics are drugs utilized for the treatment of bacterial infections and occasionally to prevent these infections.

- Some antibiotics are broad-spectrum, meaning they are effective against many types of bacteria, whereas others can only kill certain organisms
- Antibiotic use can cause allergic skin or respiratory reactions, which should be treated with antihistamines
- Other common side effects are nausea, diarrhea, and yeast infections due to disruption of normal flora
- Penicillin and most of its derivatives (e.g., amoxicillin and ampicillin) are broad-spectrum antibiotics
- In particular, ampicillin is given prophylactically and during and after invasive procedures to dental patients at risk for bacterial endocarditis
- Several penicillin derivatives (e.g., oxacillin) are given mainly for *Staphylococcus aureus* infections and Penicillin G is used only for gram-positive bacteria
- People with penicillin allergies are generally given another antibiotic called erythromycin
- Another common class of antibiotics is the tetracyclines, which can discolor emerging teeth and precipitate kidney failure

ANTICHOLINERGIC DRUGS, ANALGESICS, AND TRANQUILIZERS

Anticholinergic drugs block nerve impulses.

- They have a variety of applications
- For example, they are used to reduce lung secretions while a patient is under general anesthesia, to treat bradycardia, and to dilate the eyes
- In the context of dentistry, the most common usage for anticholinergics is the inhibition of saliva flow in order to perform activities such as the taking of an impression
- The drugs of choice in these instances are either atropine sulfate or propantheline bromide
- Any drug that relieves pain but does not cause unconsciousness is considered an analgesic
- Non-narcotic analgesics (such as ibuprofen or acetaminophen) or narcotic ones may be administered in the dental office for relief
- Aspirin is less likely to be given because it inhibits healing due to its blood-thinning and clot-suppressing qualities. It also irritates the stomach
- The narcotic analgesics morphine and codeine are discussed elsewhere
- Tranquilizers, particularly diazepam (Valium), are often given prior to procedures for relaxation

BLOOD AND BLOOD DYSCRASIAS

Blood is necessary for transportation of nutrients and other substances in the body, regulation of functions such as body temperature and pH, and protection against infection and injury.

- Blood consists mainly of the liquid plasma, which transports the various substances, and the solid cellular portion called corpuscles
- There are three types of corpuscles, erythrocytes (red blood cells containing the oxygen carrier protein hemoglobin), leukocytes (white blood cells with immune functions), and thrombocytes or platelets (involved with blood clotting)
- People with blood dyscrasias or disorders have some defect in a blood component

- The most common blood disorders are hemophilia, a hereditary defect in which blood clots slowly predisposing the individual (usually male) to extensive blood loss with the slightest injury, and leukemia, a progressive blood cancer in which abnormal leukocytes grow uncontrollably

BLOOD LOSS

Patients experiencing significant blood loss may need a donor blood transfusion.

- The blood type as well as the Rh factor status of both donor and recipient must be considered before transfusion
- The ABO system groups or types people's blood as A, B, AB, or O based on the antigen on the red blood cells (RBCs)
- Type O individuals have none of these antigens
- If an antigen is absent on the RBCs, the person will have plasma antibodies to that antigen and vice versa
- A donor must have the same blood type as the recipient or the donor must lack the recipient's RBC antigens, meaning Type O individuals are universal donors
- Conversely, type AB individuals are universal recipients
- People with Type A or B can receive their own or Type O blood but can donate only to their own or Type AB individuals
- In addition, both donor and recipient should be either Rh positive or negative
- Patients with hemophilia should be transfused as soon as possible if they have blood loss

VIRAL HEPATITIS CARRIER PRECAUTIONS

There are 5 major viruses and a number of other viruses that can cause the disease hepatitis.

- Hepatitis is inflammation of the liver
- It is also characterized by jaundice, abdominal pain, fever, and weakness
- Two types of hepatitis, Types A and E, are transient
- They are caused by contact with contaminated food or water and usually just cause temporary flu-like symptoms
- People with Type A hepatitis can be treated with gamma globulin injections or the Havrix vaccine
- Hepatitis types B, C and D are bloodborne
- Hepatitis B is quite virulent and dental personnel should be vaccinated against it with Heptavax-B, Recombivax HB or Energix B in a sequence of 3 injections
- Hepatitis C is less virulent but more chronic, and vaccine development is impeded by its mutational ability
- Both Hepatitis B and C may present asymptomatically, as jaundice, loss of appetite, abdominal discomfort, fever, muscle pain, or weakness
- Hepatitis D can only replicate in conjunction with Hepatitis B
- Personnel should use PPE and avoid contact with blood or other bodily fluids of individuals with hepatitis

HIV Carrier Precautions

The human immunodeficiency virus (HIV) is transmitted via sexual intercourse, from mother to fetus, or through contact with infected blood products.

- The virus is a retrovirus and replicates in the immune cells called T-lymphocytes
- Some HIV carriers appear asymptomatic while others have ambiguous conditions such as weight loss, fever, or diarrhea
- HIV infection may proceed to AIDS, acquired immunodeficiency syndrome, characterized by a cluster of symptoms such as pneumonia, a skin tumor called Kaposi's sarcoma, and opportunistic infections such as *Candida*
- AIDS is incurable but there are now several classes of drugs used to slow its effects, including reverse transcriptase and protease inhibitors
- The most commonly used drugs are zidovudine (AZT) and acyclovir
- Dental personnel should wear PPE and avoid contact with blood or bodily fluids of patients with HIV or AIDS

Ulcers

Many oral ulcers or sores are not contagious and can be soothed with topical anesthetics.

- Others are called cold sores and are caused by herpes simplex virus type 1 or 2 (HSV1 and HSV2)
- Herpetic lesions are vesicles filled with fluid containing virus and are quite contagious if broken
- Lip clusters of these sores are termed herpes labialis
- Herpes viruses attach to nerve cells and remain in the body for life, usually dormant but reactivated by exposure to stressors or acidic food
- The dental team should avoid contact with these cold sores and reschedule the patient, if possible, when lesions are present
- If procedures are performed, topical treatments can provide some relief
- Gloves and other PPE should be worn
- If lesions break, the dental worker can get crusty ulcerations, called herpetic willow, on his or her hands or fingers

Bacterial Endocarditis

Bacterial endocarditis is inflammation of the lining of the heart caused by a bacterial infection.

- Patients with a history of congenital heart disease or rheumatic fever are very susceptible to bacterial endocarditis
- People who have undergone open heart surgery (e.g., heart valve replacement), joint replacements, or organ transplants are also predisposed to development of bacterial endocarditis
- An individual with a heart murmur is at risk for endocarditis
- Insertion of dental implants also puts patients at risk
- Any patient with any of these risk factors should be given a broad spectrum antibiotic prior to dental treatments or procedures to avoid infection

Patient Education and Office Management

Patient Education

PREVENTIVE DENTISTRY COMPONENTS

Good preventive dentistry is multifaceted.

- It involves daily brushing and flossing for removal of plaque and bacteria
- Correct techniques for brushing and flossing should be used
- It is advisable to use a disclosing agent at regular intervals to see how successful the removal has been
- Children who are still developing dentition should undergo a fluoride program, including treatments at the office and in the home
- The individual should make routine visits to the dentist
- These visits should include an examination, cleaning, and dental procedures if indicated
- In addition, good nutrition and adequate exercise have a positive impact on general health, including health of teeth and bones

MAINTENANCE OF ORAL HEALTH

The oral health of infants is the responsibility of the parent or another adult.

- The adult removes the infant's plaque with an infant toothbrush or cloth while the child reclines
- The preschool years are the time when the child is first brought to the dentist (about 3 years old) and introduced to toothbrushes and other oral hygiene
- At these ages, children respond to visual instruction, but they also have a short attention span
- Role-playing can help to teach the child oral hygiene habits, but the parent should oversee or perform the tooth brushing at bedtime
- Children ages 5 to 8 have a longer attention span and are eager for knowledge
- They can be taught good oral hygiene techniques with visual aids like short videos or pictures
- Older children, from about age 9 to 12, have an even longer attention span, greater curiosity, and the ability to brush and floss effectively on their own
- They also have unique issues, such as peer group acceptance and dealing with mixed dentition, which the dental assistant should keep in mind when providing instruction

TEENAGERS, ADULTS, AND OLDER ADULTS

Peer pressure and concern about personal appearance are motivating factors for the actions of all teenagers.

- Younger teenagers, about 13 to 15 years old, often have poor coordination (due to growth spurts) and bad eating habits, therefore, they often have trouble with practices like flossing, and the decay rate in this age group increases dramatically
- The dental assistant should give individualized instruction and encouragement to motivate young teenagers
- Older teenagers (ages 16 to 19) have similar issues, but they also tend to question authority and have increasing demands on their time

133

- The assistant needs to act more as a friend
- Explaining the processes involved in plaque and caries formation is a useful strategy
- Young and middle-aged adults should be approached on an individualized basis and included in their oral health decisions
- Once they reach about age 60, some patients will have age-related concerns, such as retaining teeth, disease-specific difficulties in maintaining oral hygiene, or the use of drugs that interfere with oral health
- The professional needs to give advice based on each specific case

ORAL HYGIENE AIDS

Oral hygiene aids include disclosing agents, dentifrice, toothbrushes, flosses, mouth rinses, chewing gum, and a variety of interdental aids.

- Dentifrice is another term for toothpaste used by the patient with a toothbrush or floss
- Dentifrice products earn the ADA Seal of Acceptance if they are deemed to be both safe and effective
- Toothpastes contain abrasive materials and often fluoride for decay prevention or other ingredients (for example whiteners or calculus inhibitors)
- Mouth rinses are designed to be swirled in the mouth to dislodge debris or temporarily get rid of halitosis as adjuncts to brushing and flossing
- Some have ingredients that eradicate microorganisms as well
- Special oral hygiene chewing gums are used after eating carbohydrates to encourage saliva production and loosen debris
- Interdental aids are designed to assist in cleaning between the teeth and to stimulate the gums
- They include the interproximal brush, dental stimulators, floss holders and threaders, the water irrigation device (all discussed on another card)
- Disclosing agents, toothbrushes and flosses are discussed elsewhere

VARIOUS INTERDENTAL AIDS

Interproximal brushes consist of a handle (often bent) attached to a small, nylon-bristled brush.

- They are used to reach into interproximal or open bi- or trifurcation areas or under orthodontic brackets
- Dental stimulators are used to stimulate the soft tissues in interproximal areas and get rid of plaque
- Numerous toothbrushes have the rubber tip version on the opposite end of the brush
- Alternatively, there are wooden dental stimulators made of balsam wedges and plastic handles with toothpick tips attached; both should be moistened before use
- Floss holders are apparatuses shaped like a "Y" that hold floss for easy access to different interproximal areas
- The floss is shifted up and down on the side of the tooth and into the sulcus
- Floss threaders are made of rigid plastic shaped into a large loop at one end through which floss is threaded
- The straight end is inserted into one side of the space and pulled out the other for removal, leaving the floss for elimination of plaque and debris
- A water irrigation device uses pulses of water to remove debris
- These devices are mostly used with orthodontic brackets and prostheses and are not effective against plaque

TOOTHBRUSHES

All toothbrushes fall into two main categories: manual or mechanical.

- Manual toothbrushes usually consist of a head containing the bristles, an indented shank adjacent to the head, and a longer handle
- There may also be a rubber dental stimulator on the end
- The head has a toe end at the exterior and a heel end
- Bristle configurations differ on various brushes; they are usually spaced or multi-tufted
- Manual toothbrushes with soft, nylon bristles are advocated because they are durable and will not wear away the teeth or gums
- Mechanical toothbrushes are attached in some way to a recharging unit
- They have heads that can be moved in various directions
- Motion options can include reciprocating (back and forth), vibratory (quick back and forth), orbital (circular), arched (in a semi-circle), elliptical (oval rotation), or some combination of these movements
- Mechanical toothbrushes may also include sonic action

MANUAL TOOTH BRUSHING TECHNIQUES

The main objective of tooth brushing is the thorough cleaning of every surface of all teeth.

- With manual brushing this should take 2 to 3 minutes
- Manual brushing techniques include the Bass, modified Bass, Charter, modified Stillman, rolling stroke, and modified scrub brushing techniques
- Dentists most often recommend the Bass or modified Bass techniques
- With the Bass technique, the toothbrush bristles are slanted at 45 degrees to the teeth toward the gingival sulcus
- Small areas are sequentially brushed for a count of 10 each with small back and forth movements
- The lingual surfaces of the front teeth are cleaned using the toe bristles
- The modified Bass technique is essentially the same except after each area has been cleaned the bristles are brought up over the crown toward the biting surface
- Bass techniques are effective at removing plaque near the gums

CHARTERS AND MODIFIED SCRUB BRUSHING TECHNIQUES

These brushing techniques are effective for plaque removal and gum stimulation.

- With the Charters brushing technique, the toothbrush head is pointed toward the end of the root
- The brushes touch the gingival centered between adjacent teeth and are aimed toward the teeth
- Small areas are sequentially brushed for a count of 10 each with small back and forth movements
- Front teeth are brushed with the sides of the toe bristles and the brush parallel to the teeth
- The modified scrub brushing technique uses back-and-forth movements centered initially between the gum and tooth
- The brush is held perpendicular to the tooth surface
- This is repeated until all teeth have been cleaned

MODIFIED STILLMAN AND ROLLING STROKE BRUSHING TECHNIQUES

These brushing techniques are effective for plaque removal and gingival stimulation.

- In both, the initial position of the bristles is toward the apex of the tooth
- The modified Stillman method also positions the handle level with the biting surface
- The bristles are brushed downward simultaneously with a back-and-forth action to cover the complete surface of the tooth
- This is done for a count of 10 to a minimum of 5 sequences before continuing to the next tooth and repeating the sequence
- With the rolling stroke brushing technique, the toothbrush is held parallel to the tooth with the bristles toward the apex
- The bristles are rolled from the gums down toward the teeth including the biting surface
- Each tooth is brushed in this manner 5 times before moving to the next one
- A similar motion is applied on the lingual surfaces of the front teeth, using either the toe or heel portion

DENTAL FLOSS AND FLOSSING TECHNIQUE

Dental flossing removes plaque and fragments from proximal surfaces of teeth.

- Traditional dental floss comes as a thread that is either unwaxed or waxed
- Waxed floss glides more easily and is less likely to tear or snag
- Flosses come in many varieties: flat tape, finely textured, colored, and flavored
- Flossing should be done using about 18 inches of floss
- The ends are secured around the middle and ring fingers of each hand, and a short section (about an inch) is grasped between the thumb and index finger of each hand
- The floss is drawn into each proximal space, using a gentle back-and-forth motion
- In the maxilla, both thumbs or a thumb and finger should be used, and for the mandible, the two index fingers are suggested
- The floss should be wrapped around the proximal surface and into part of the sulcus
- The floss is moved up and down along the surface for plaque removal, transferred to the proximal surface of the adjoining tooth, and the action repeated
- A new section of floss should be used for each space
- Flossing should include the distal surface of the last molar

SPECIAL NEEDS PATIENTS

All patients with special needs require empathy and individual attention from the dental professional.

- The nausea that usually accompanies pregnancy presents problems related to oral hygiene
- Acid regurgitated from the stomach during bouts of nausea promotes decay; the act of tooth brushing often causes gagging, and pregnant women commonly have bleeding gums
- Pregnant women should be made aware of this, and dental hygiene should be done at times when they are not nauseous
- Cancer patients commonly experience xerostomia or unusual mouth dryness, widespread caries (including the roots), gum bleeding, and deficient muscle function
- Approaches to oral hygiene issues include use of topical fluoride and/or extra-soft or foam toothbrushes
- Patients with heart disease commonly experience similar problems
- Patients with arthritis may need to use special large toothbrushes or floss holders

CARIOGENIC FOODS

Carbohydrates contain the chemical elements carbon, hydrogen, and oxygen, and are comprised of sugars, starches, and fibers.

- Carbohydrates are found in natural sources such as fruits, grains, and legumes
- In most cases, these naturally-occurring carbohydrates are not broken down to simple sugars until they arrive at the stomach
- Cariogenic foods are ones that are converted to simple sugars right in the mouth where bacteria can change them into acids
- The acid eventually causes demineralization of the enamel, predisposing the teeth to caries or decay
- Manufactured sweets such as candies and soft drinks as well as some naturally-occurring ones like raisins and certain fruits do stick to the teeth and are cariogenic
- The dental assistant should evaluate the patient's diet for use of cariogenic foods and the possible consequences
- The acid from these foods can be somewhat neutralized if they are eaten with other types of food stimulating saliva production
- Conversely, eating them late at night when saliva production is low enhances cariogenic potential
- New teeth in infants are susceptible to nursing bottle syndrome, rampant decay due to liquid sweets such as fruit juice

SOURCES OF ENERGY

Anything consumed by an individual is his diet.

- Nutrients are chemical substances in the diet that are essential for growth, maintenance, and healing
- Nutrients fall into 6 general categories
- Three of these are potential sources of energy: carbohydrates, fats, and proteins
- The other 3 classifications are vitamins, minerals, and water
- Carbohydrates (sugars, starches and fibers) primarily provide energy
- They should comprise at least half of an individual's diet
- Fats and their constituent lipids are water-insoluble and contain fatty acids
- Fat is used for insulation, transport of certain vitamins, and as a source of energy when sugars are inaccessible
- Proteins are complex compounds made up of linked amino acids
- They are provided in plant and animal sources, and are vital for cell growth and repair
- Of 20 possible amino acids, 10 are considered essential and must be provided in the diet
- Animal proteins like eggs or milk contain all the essential amino acids and are complete, whereas many plant sources do not and are considered incomplete
- If different incomplete foods are eaten at the same time, they can be complementary

CALORIE CONSUMPTION AND EXPENDITURE

Calories consumed provide energy. Carbohydrates supply 4 Calories (C or Cal) per gram consumed, fats 9 Cal/gram, and proteins 4 Cal/gram.

- A person's rate of metabolism is the relationship between bodily changes and energy expenditure
- Everyone has a resting or basal metabolic rate (BMR). BMR is generally higher in children, thin people, and expectant women
- While the primary energy source is carbohydrates, fats are also utilized when sugars are inaccessible
- Conversely, if calories are not used, they are converted to fat and stored
- Both carbohydrates and fatty acids comprising fats are made of the elements carbon, oxygen, and hydrogen in different configurations

FAT-SOLUBLE VITAMINS

Nutrients that carry out various essential functions are called vitamins.

- They are not energy sources
- Four vitamins are fat-soluble and retained in the liver and other fatty tissues, vitamins A, D, E, and K
- Vitamin A is available in the form of carotene in dark leafy vegetables and orange or yellow fruits and from animal sources such as dairy products and liver
- It is essential for maintenance of mucous membranes, bones, skin (epithelial tissue), and vision
- Vitamin D or cholecalciferol is necessary for good bone and tooth growth
- It is available in animal sources such as eggs, liver, and fortified milk
- It can also be produced in the body after ultraviolet ray or sun exposure
- Vitamin E or alpha-tocopherol is obtained from plant sources, such as margarines or salad dressings
- It acts as an antioxidant to prevent other nutrients from breaking down
- Vitamin K is also supplied in green leafy vegetables and animal products such as milk, liver, and egg yolks
- Its primary function is to stimulate the formation of prothrombin, which is involved in blood clotting and coagulation

WATER-SOLUBLE VITAMINS

Vitamin C and vitamin B complex vitamins are water-soluble.

- Vitamin C or ascorbic acid is found in all citrus fruits and vegetables such as tomatoes and broccoli
- Vitamin C is a necessary component of collagen needed in connective tissue; it prevents scurvy, aids in wound healing, and helps tooth development
- There are numerous vitamin B complex vitamins, all with different utilities
- They include the following: thiamin (B_1), essential as a coenzyme in the oxidation of glucose and to avert the degenerative nerve disease beriberi; riboflavin (B_2), which aids growth, energy release from food, and protein production; and niacin or nicotinic acid, which is utilized in ATP synthesis and thwarts gastrointestinal and nervous system troubles
- These 3 play roles in energy production

- Other B complex vitamins include the following: pyridoxine (B_6), which plays a role in the production of antibodies, nonessential amino acids, and niacin; vitamin B_{12}, used to synthesize red blood cells (RBCs) and to maintain myelin sheaths; folacin, essential for RBC production; and biotin and pantothenic acid, which both function primarily in energy metabolism

EXCESS VITAMIN INTAKE

All vitamins have beneficial effects in proper amounts.

- Deficiencies of any vitamin can have a detrimental effect
- Examples include night blindness or inadequate bone growth for vitamin A, rickets and inadequately developed teeth for vitamin D, mouth fissures and inflammation of the tongue with deficits of either vitamin B_2 or B_6, and scurvy or muscle cramps for vitamin C
- Deficits in a number of vitamins can result in blood problems such as RBC destruction with a vitamin E deficiency or pernicious anemia with a vitamin B_{12} deficit
- Conversely, many vitamins are toxic if consumed in too large a quantity
- This is true for all of the fat-soluble vitamins
- For example, toxic amounts of vitamin A can cause such things as stunted growth and termination of menstruation
- Vitamin D toxicity can result in kidney stones
- Vitamin E toxicity can cause hypertension
- Vitamin K toxicity can cause hemolytic anemia or jaundice
- High amounts of many water-soluble vitamins are not toxic because they are excreted in the urine
- Only excessive amounts of vitamins C, B_6, and niacin have potential toxicities
- For example, vitamin C in excess can cause kidney stones

MAJOR MINERALS

Minerals are elements that cannot be broken down chemically. In the body, there are 7 major elements found in larger quantities than a number of other trace elements.

- Minerals that are found as negatively or positively charged ions are termed electrolytes
- Two of the major minerals, calcium and phosphorus, are important for development of bones and teeth and are necessary to prevent osteoporosis
- Each also has other functions
- Calcium is involved in muscle contraction, conduction of nerve impulses, and blood clotting
- Phosphorus is involved in energy transfer and pH balance
- Milk and cheese are good sources of each
- Sodium and potassium are major minerals that are complementary to one another in maintenance of fluid balance in the blood
- Sodium is found in table salt and many foods and can cause high blood pressure in excess
- Table salt also contains the mineral chlorine, which has a number of roles including pH balance
- Sulfur is important because it is a necessary component of protein and also plays a role in metabolism of energy
- Magnesium, found mostly in green vegetables and whole grains, also affects energy metabolism

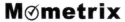

DIETARY TRACE MINERALS

A number of minerals are found in the body in small or trace amounts.

- Fluorine, which is necessary for strong teeth and to avert osteoporosis, is considered a trace element
- Numerous trace minerals facilitate metabolic processes, including iodine, copper, chromium, selenium, manganese, and molybdenum
- Iodine is unique in that is concentrated in the thyroid gland
- The trace mineral iron is a carrier of oxygen in blood; a deficit of iron can cause anemia
- Cobalt is also necessary for red blood cell maintenance
- Zinc is utilized in the immune system and promotes tissue growth

Office Operations

DENTAL JURISPRUDENCE, CONTRACTS AND TORTS

Jurisprudence is the legal system set up and enforced at various governmental levels.

- Those laws that pertain to dentistry are referred to as dental jurisprudence
- There are both civil and criminal laws
- Civil laws are more often invoked in the dental setting as they pertain to either contracts or torts
- A contract is an enforceable covenant between two or more competent individuals
- An agreement between a dentist and his or her patient is a contract
- It can be an expressed contract in which terms are established in writing or verbally or it can be an implied contract in which necessary actions create the contract
- Tort law governs the other branch of civil law
- Torts, which relate more to standard of care, are wrongful actions that end up causing injury to the other person
- Criminal laws speak to crimes recognized as endangering society in general
- There are occasions when criminal law may apply in dentistry, usually resulting in fines, incarceration, and/or actions from the state dentistry board

CONTRACT LAW

There is an expressed or more often an implied contract between the dentist and patient.

- The dental assistant or other personnel are considered agents of the dentist who is ultimately responsible for breach of contract under the Doctrine of Respondeat Superior
- Nevertheless, the assistant's words or actions regarding care are legally binding upon the dentist
- A breach of contract is failure to fulfill and complete its terms
- There are only four types of situations where a contract can be legally abandoned:
  - These are when the patient releases the dentist by failure to return
  - When the patient does not comply with specific instructions from the dentist regarding care
  - If the patient no longer requires treatment
  - If the dentist formally withdraws from the case, in this situation, the dentist should send a certified letter to the patient explaining the situation to preclude any charges of patient abandonment. A certified letter from dentist to patient is also suggested when the latter is discharged

STANDARD CARE LEGAL ASPECTS

Issues related to standard of care are generally covered by tort laws.

- Dental specialists are expected to provide due care, the accepted reasonable and judicious care
- Malpractice is professional misconduct resulting in failure to provide due care
- Most malpractice lawsuits are related to professional negligence, the failure to perform what is considered standard care
- Tort laws also pertain to what is considered unethical or immoral behavior by the professional resulting in harm to the patient

- The main examples are defamation of character, invasion of privacy, fraud, assault, and battery
- Defamation of character is harm to another individual's character, name, or reputation through untrue and malicious statements, either written (libel) or spoken (slander)
- Invasion of privacy is unsolicited or unauthorized exposure of patient information
- Fraud is intentional dishonesty for unfair or illegal gain
- Assault is the declaration of intent of inappropriate touching of a patient and battery is the actual act of touching
- People who provide unpaid assistance to the injured in emergency situations are protected under the Good Samaritan Law

THE AMERICANS WITH DISABILITIES ACT

In 1990, the Americans with Disabilities Act was federally passed.

- It mandates that people with disabilities cannot be discriminated against in terms of employment and access to public services, accommodations, and goods
- It also made provisions for more sophisticated telecommunication services to facilitate the hearing and speech impaired
- The terms of this Act translate into the requirements for dental offices to have ramps, entryways, and treatment rooms that provide access and accommodate the needs of the disabled
- There must be at least one room where patients in wheelchairs can be positioned for dental procedures
- Technically the Act applies to facilities with more than 15 employees, but all offices should strive to comply

PATIENT'S DENTAL RECORDS

A patient's dental record should be correct and current.

- All care and payments should be documented legibly in ink
- Corrections can be made, but a line must be struck through the original entry, and the new information must be initialed and dated
- Dental records can legally be subpoenaed by a court as can the professional
- Records should be kept pretty much indefinitely because the statute of limitations, the time period for local legal action, varies
- A signed informed consent form should also be in the chart for any surgical procedures
- A professional must explain the procedure, risks, expected results, alternatives, and perils associated with denying treatment before asking the patient to sign the informed consent form
- Implied consent is an implicit contract that occurs between dentist and patient whenever the latter allows work to be done

DENTISTRY ETHICS

Ethics are sets of moral principles or values indicative of the times.

- Dental ethics are spelled out in The American Dental Association Principles of Ethics
- The main ethical concerns related to the practice of dentistry relate to advertising, professional fees and other charges, and the responsibilities and entitlements of the dentist relative to the patient

- In today's world, dental advertising is considered to be perfectly ethical as long as it is truthful, but years ago it was more eschewed
- Ethical behavior related to professional fees and charges means that these confirm to what is charged locally, the correct charge is billed, and things like insurance dealings and missed appointments can be charged
- Current ethics dictate that the dentist must not discriminate against seeing a patient on any basis like race, religion, or even HIV status. HIV-infected dentists must limit their work to procedures and techniques that will not infect others
- It is considered unethical for the dentist to be swayed by financial gains

HIPAA

HIPAA is the Health Insurance Portability and Accountability Act of 1996.

- It was ratified to institute safeguards related to electronically-conveyed healthcare communications
- These dealings include claims, transfer of funds, and eligibility and claims status inquiries and replies
- The Act also directed the Department of Health and Human Services (HHS) to implement national standards for clerical and financial electronic transmissions related to healthcare
- Dentists as well as other healthcare providers and health plans must be in compliance at this time
- The areas covered in the HIPAA related to privacy standards include protected health information, the individual's rights, the latest guidelines for dental offices, parameters related to use and disclosure, enforcement, and preemption

HIPAA PHI PARAMETERS

Protected health information (PHI) is any knowledge that can or possibly could distinguish a patient.

- If the information contains any potential identifying factors such as name, Social Security number, birth date, etc., it must be guarded
- This means, for example, that in a dental office all records should be covered up (or locked up if unattended), phone conversations should be discrete, computers and fax machines should be out of patient viewing areas
- Patient information that has been transformed in some way that the individual cannot be identified can be openly transmitted
- Each dental office is required to have a privacy officer (PO) who is responsible for informing patients about their privacy rights
- HIPAA grants patients the right to access and copy their own dental information
- Each dental office is required to have a written PHI policy, including requirements for use and disclosure of patient information and procedures for handling grievances
- Information release to third parties must be authorized by the patient and kept to a minimum
- Violations of PHI under HIPAA are punishable by up to $250,000 in fines and 10 years imprisonment

DENTAL STAFF MANUAL IN COMPLIANCE WITH HIPAA

There are a number of minimum requirements about what must be included in dental staff manuals under HIPAA.

- A dental staff manual should specify a privacy officer (PO) in charge of informing patients about their privacy rights
- It should also include the job descriptions of all personnel
- There should be a privacy policy statement
- The manual should contain a HIPAA training plan with training dates
- A number of forms related to HIPAA compliance, documentation, and the scheme for reporting of violations should be incorporated
- Confidentiality agreements between the dentist and patient should be available
- The agreements that the office has with business associates, such as dental laboratories or computer services, should be included
- There should also be wording about the contents and the contingencies for change

ADAA CODE OF PROFESSIONAL CONDUCT

There are 17 pledges that members of the American Dental Assistants Association (ADAA) subscribe to in their Code of Professional Conduct.

- The pledges are primarily related to ethics
- Many of these relate to the relationship between the dental assistant and the Association, such as:
  - abiding by the bylaws
  - maintaining loyalty to the Association
  - following the Association's objectives
  - maintaining respect for and serving the members and employees
  - adhering to the Association's regulations
  - refraining from spreading malicious information regarding the ADAA
  - utilizing sound business principles related to the organization
  - acting cooperatively with staff and members
  - being of service to the Association
  - instilling public confidence in the Association
  - the member also pledges to uphold high personal standards of conduct
  - separate personal opinions from those endorsed by the ADAA
  - refrain from acceptance of compensation from other members
  - a statement about influencing relevant legislation in a legal and ethical way is also included

OPENING THE OFFICE

Every morning the dental assistant is responsible turning on lights, dental units, the vacuum system, the air compressor, equipment associated with radiographic processing, sterilizing equipment, the communication system, and the computers.

- The assistant should do housekeeping chores such as unlocking files, organizing the reception and business areas, replenishing water and solutions if necessary, for radiographic processing, preparing disinfecting solutions, setting out trays and lab work for the first patients, and restocking any necessary supplies

- The assistant should change into protective clothing such as a lab coat or uniform
- The assistant should also check the patient schedule and finish any overnight sterilization procedures

CLOSING THE OFFICE

One or more dental assistants participate in closing the office every day.

- The assistant must clean the chairs and units in the treatment rooms, flush various systems, and shut off switches
- Radiographs should be processed, mounted and filed and radiographic processing equipment and the safe light should be turned off
- Used instruments should be sterilized
- Trays for the next day should be set up
- The assistant should check whether all laboratory work has been sent there and earlier work has been sent back
- The assistant should deal with assigned chores such as insurance, bookkeeping, and confirming and pulling charts for the next day's appointments
- The assistant should turn off all business equipment, turn on the answering machine, bolt windows and doors, and change out of his or her uniform into regular clothes before leaving

TREATMENT ROOM PREPARATION

The dental assistant is responsible for preparing the treatment room between patients.

- This includes cleaning, disinfecting, and placing barriers on all areas (including charts) that may be touched
- The Infection Control (ICE) exam covers appropriate procedures
- The rheostat, chairs, and mobile carts are pulled out of the patient's pathway, and the dental light is lifted up
- The dental chair should be about 15 to 18 inches above the floor with the arm positioned for patient access
- The dental assistant should review the chart and set out any needed radiographs, trays, or lab work

GREETING AND PREPARING THE DENTAL PATIENT

After preparing the treatment room, the assistant greets the patient by name in the reception area and escorts the patient to the treatment room.

- The assistant illustrates where to put personal items
- The assistant may offer mouthwash to the patient, and then he or she seats the patient in the dental chair
- Tissues for lipstick removal, lip lubricants, and a drink of water are usually offered at this time
- The dental assistant puts the napkin or bib on the patient and gives the patient safety glasses to wear
- The assistant should appraise the medical history for changes, inquire whether the patient has any questions, and place radiographs on the view box
- The patient is then positioned for treatment
- This involves placing the patient in the supine position with the head supported by the headrest

- The rheostat, operator's stool, assistant's stool, and lamp are positioned
- The assistant dons a mask and protective eyewear
- After washing his or her hands the assistant dons gloves as well
- The assistant then sets up trays, the saliva ejector, the air-water syringe, evacuator, and handpieces

DENTAL PATIENT DISMISSAL

After the operator has finished the dental procedure, the dental assistant is responsible for rinsing and evacuating the patient's mouth.

- The assistant pulls the dental light aside, positions the dental chair to upright, removes fragments on the patient's face, and takes off the bib
- The patient is instructed to stay seated for a minute in case he or she is woozy
- The used bib, evacuator and air-water syringe tips, and saliva ejector are removed and put on the tray
- The assistant then either takes off the treatment gloves and washes his or her hands or uses overgloves to immediately record procedures performed on the chart or electronically
- The chart and radiographs are collected
- The patient is provided with postoperative instructions and his or her personal items and is taken back by the assistant to the receptionist who deals with later appointments and payments

DENTAL RECEPTIONIST AND DENTAL OFFICE BOOKKEEPER

The dental receptionist is responsible for initially greeting patients, helping them to fill out needed paperwork, answering the telephone, taking memos, arranging appointments, overseeing the charts and records, and other assigned tasks.

- The receptionist may or may not assume the role of dental office bookkeeper
- The employee hired to be the dental office bookkeeper deals with all office finances, including accounts receivable and accounts payable
- Usually accounts receivable or money owed to the practice is dealt with in a bookkeeping system different from the one for accounts payable for which the office owes money
- The bookkeeper may also handle dental insurance or payment arrangement details or the inventory and supply system
- Many dental offices may have an office manager who may assume some of these roles

TELEPHONE ETIQUETTE

Calls are usually answered initially by the receptionist in the dental office, but all personnel should be aware of good telephone etiquette and techniques.

- The receptionist should be ready to answer all incoming calls within 2 to 3 rings
- The receptionist's demeanor should make it clear to the caller that the receptionist is organized, attentive, and courteous
- Anyone in charge of answering the phone should speak clearly and directly into the mouthpiece, pronouncing words properly and speaking at a normal speed
- People answering the phone should also practice good listening skills, including obtaining and using the caller's name
- The receptionist screens the call to figure out to whom it should be directed

- The receptionist often must take a message, including date, time, caller, the caller's phone number, who the message is for, the communication, and callback parameters
- If it is necessary to place a caller on hold, that delay should be short, no more than one minute
- Outgoing calls should consist primarily of next day confirmations of appointments
- When communicating with patients whose primary language is not English, patience, repetition, speaking slowly at a normal volume, and sometimes an interpreter are indicated

OFFICE COMMUNICATION TECHNOLOGIES

Current communication technologies have to an extent changed the way some dental offices operate.

- There should always be a means of access to dental personnel in the advent of an emergency
- Today that can mean answering machines that are turned on when personnel are not present and checked upon return, answering services manned by individuals who can contact the dentist, and voice mail systems that automatically route the individual to a mailbox that takes a message for a specific professional
- The professional may be contacted via a beeper or other paging system that alerts him or her to call a particular patient's number
- Increasingly the patient and/or healthcare professional may carry a cellular phone to send and receive calls
- Written communications and data can be transmitted via a facsimile on a fax machine
- Electronic mail (e-mail) has made it possible to digitally receive, store, send, and forward messages

DENTAL BUSINESS OFFICE COMPUTERIZATION

These days most dental business office systems are at least partially computerized.

- Desktop personal computers or PCs are most often used as the physical equipment or hardware
- The software that is most applicable is word processing, graphics, and database management programs and spreadsheets
- Software packages such as Microsoft Works often combine all of these functions
- Database management is particularly important in a dental office because these programs can store vital patient contact and insurance information
- The other programs are useful for grouping and analyzing of data
- Access to email and the World Wide Web are increasingly necessary as well

COMPUTER SAFETY ISSUES

The office computers must be safeguarded against computer viruses through installation of a program.

- Information should also be backed up every day on a disc or external hard drive
- In terms of the computer operator, practice of good ergonomics or workplace design is the central concern
- For example, the computer monitor should be positioned with the top just below eye level and at a slight backward incline
- The keyboard should be placed at a height that allows for relaxed shoulders and flat wrists

- The computer chair should be designed such that the seat back supports the lower back
- The armrests should be low enough that they are not used during keyboard use
- The seat should be shallow enough to permit sitting back
- The person should be seated with the thighs at the height of or just above the knees, feet firmly planted on the floor, and head directly over the shoulders
- Eye glare should be prevented with screen glare protectors, and eye fatigue should be addressed by looking away from the computer 10 minutes for every hour in front of the screen

PATIENT SCHEDULING

Patient scheduling is usually done by the receptionist, either in an appointment book or on the computer.

- There are various formats and color-coding schemes for appointment books
- Ten- or sometimes 15-minute units of time are usually blocked out for expected procedures
- This generally includes some time with the dental assistant alone in addition to time with the dentist, allowing for double booking when one professional is free to attend to another patient's needs
- The outline of dates when the dentist is available throughout the year can be set out on an appointment matrix
- Buffer times can be set aside for dental emergencies
- Children should be scheduled around nap times or school hours and considerations should be made for patients with special conditions or needs
- Increasing patient scheduling is done using computer software

APPOINTMENT BOOK ENTRIES

An appropriate time should be determined in conjunction with the patient.

- All appointment book entries should be made in pencil to allow for changes
- The patient's name, phone number, age (for children), and type and length of appointment should be indicated
- The patient is immediately given an appointment card
- The receptionist scheduling the appointment should be familiar enough with the length of various proceeds to avoid scheduling problems like unscheduled down time, overtime in which procedures take longer than scheduled, or overlap of time in which one of the professionals needs to be in two places at once or more than one patient is scheduled for the same treatment room simultaneously
- The entries in the appointment book or one the computer are often used to set up a daily schedule illustrating blocks of time each dentist will see certain patients that day, the patient's phone number, and procedures to be performed

PATIENT RECALL SYSTEMS

Patients are usually scheduled for continued care or recall appointments by one of 4 methods.

- Computer recall involves immediately placing information into a computer program after a patient appointment with a recall time frame indicated
- Toward the end of each month, the computer generates a listing of patients for recall the next month who are then contacted

- Another method is to immediately schedule the recall in the appointment book months in advance at the time the patient is in the office
- The patient is generally required to confirm the appointment when the scheduled date nears
- Another system is to have the individual fill out an addressed postcard that is filed by month and then sent to the patient a couple weeks before ideal recall; this is called a chronological card file
- The last recall system is fairly similar
- It uses a color-tagged card file system in which an index card with all pertinent patient information is kept and color tags are attached according to indicated month for recall

DENTAL RECORDS MANAGEMENT

Dental records are generally kept in file-folders (often color-coded) that are put in easily accessible file cabinets.

- The most popular type of file cabinet used in dental offices is the open-shelf lateral file cabinet, in which files can be pulled out for access
- Vertical file cabinets are often used
- Whatever type of storage is used, the files must be sorted alphabetically starting with the last name and, if necessary, proceeding to the first name and in some instances, the middle name
- File cabinets must be locked when unattended to maintain patient record confidentiality
- Patient information contained in or sent via computer or facsimile must also protect confidentiality
- Records are usually kept indefinitely, sometimes requiring other means of storage such as microfilm
- It is also suggested that the office have a so-called tickler file containing index cards with tasks that should be completed by a certain time; there are computer programs with similar files

PATIENT FEES

Dental offices set up a fee schedule for specific services rendered.

- Fees charged are defined as usual, reasonable, or customary
- The usual fee is that normally charged by the dentist
- A reasonable fee is one falling in the midrange of charges based on the procedure and difficulty
- The customary fee reflects local averages up to the 90th percentile
- Insurance companies will not reimburse amounts above what they have determined to be usual, reasonable, and customary
- When a dentist charges less, such as in instances where he or she extends professional courtesy or participates in certain insurance programs, there is no source to recover the rest of the usual, reasonable, or customary fee

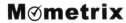

ACCOUNTS RECEIVABLE BOOKKEEPING

The dental office bookkeeper handles accounts receivable and payable.

- He or she will use either a computer system of account management or the manual pegboard system of patient account management for accounts receivable
- Computerized systems have all pertinent patient information, description of services, charges, payments, and insurance information in organized and easily accessible form
- The account status can be viewed or printed out
- The pegboard system uses day sheets that list patient names and all procedures and charges and receipts for that day
- No-carbon-required paper is used
- There are columns for balancing all daily as well as individual patient accounts receivable
- Total amounts received daily should be deposited promptly in a bank account
- Patients are usually invoiced monthly
- Partial or deferred arrangements may be extended to patients with good credit ratings

DENTAL INSURANCE CONCEPTS

A person who has contracted dental insurance is referred to as a subscriber and anyone covered by the policy is a beneficiary.

- Insurance can be primary or secondary depending on whether it is obtained via a subscriber or spouse
- Plans offered to a large number of people, usually through an employer, are group plans; individual plans are also available
- Dependents are defined as children also covered, generally less than 18 years old or still completing their full-time education
- A carrier is the insurance company administering the plan
- Carriers generally have maximum amounts they will reimburse for the year and deductible amounts before which benefits accrue
- Predetermination of benefits refers to a process by which the dentist sends a proposed treatment plan to the carrier to figure out how much will be covered

DENTAL INSURANCE ALTERNATIVES

Health maintenance organizations (HMOs) usually administer capitation programs where the dentist gets a fixed fee based on the number of patients.

- Medicare is an example of a contract fee schedule plan in which dentists in the plan agree to consent to defined and usually reduced fees for specific services
- Managed care plans focus on preventive care and limit the procedures that can be done or medications that can be prescribed
- Direct reimbursement plans do not use an insurance carrier as a middleman; here the patient pays directly for services, and then is refunded the money spent by his or her employer who is the plan administrator

DENTAL INSURANCE CLAIMS

Each procedure performed is assigned a 5-digit CDT code beginning with a D for dental.

- CDT codes are described in the ADA's *Current Dental Terminology*
- The patient must endorse on the claim form his or her assignment of benefits, which states that the benefits should be paid from the insurance carrier directly to the dentist or other provider
- Otherwise, it is tacit that patients will pay for services themselves
- Alternatively, a signature on file can be used for assignment of benefits
- The patient should also sign another area for release of information to the carrier
- There are also areas for patient identification
- Insurance claims can generally be submitted by mail or electronically
- Carriers generally have established schedules of benefits detailing amounts they will reimburse for various activities

ACCOUNTS PAYABLE

Accounts payable responsibilities are generally handed by the bookkeeper, but some functions such as inventory supply and control are often assigned to the dental assistant.

- The total amount of accounts receivable is the practice's gross income
- Accounts payable or money to be paid out for various expenses are deducted from the gross income to determine the net income or profit
- Permanent salaries, mortgage payments, and certain utilities are steady fixed expenses
- Monthly expenses that change, such as supplies or needed repairs, are variable expenses
- The combination of fixed and variable expenses is the practice's overhead
- Periodically, usually once or twice monthly, the dentist authorizes payment of certain accounts payable
- There may be a small amount of petty cash kept in the office as well

INVENTORY SUPPLIES

The dental assistant often is the person who orders supplies.

- Supplies are divided into two categories, expendable ones that are disposable and quickly consumed and non-expendable ones that are enduring and purchased only rarely
- A number of parameters affect ordering of supplies
- Each has a specific shelf life or time at which it should no longer be used or stored
- There are several considerations regarding price
- Supplies generally have a single item price, a unit price for groupings of an item, and a bulk price
- Bulk price refers to a cut-rate price available if a minimum number of units are purchased, and a price break is the smallest number of units needed to obtain a bulk price
- When ordering supplies, the buyer needs to consider the rate of use of the supply, the amount generally utilized per time period, and the lead time or interval between ordering and receipt of the product
- These two concepts are combined to determine a reorder point at which a supply needs to be bought in order to ensure continued availability

Reordering Supplies

Two of the most common methods of reordering supplies are the red flag reorder tag system and the electronic bar code system.

- In the red flag reorder tag system, a tag is affixed to an item in inventory at the previously identified reorder point
- At minimum, the name of the supply is on the tag
- When the product has gotten down to the reorder point, the tag is removed and put in a specified area for all needed reordering
- Every type of supply has an index card with information needed for ordering
- The tag is attached to the upper-right corner when the item should be ordered, the left-hand corner after ordering, and removed upon receipt
- New inventory is placed in the back of the pile and the red tag reaffixed at the new reorder point
- With an electronic bar code system, supplies that need to be reordered are identified by a specific bar code that is kept in a book
- A bar code wand is swept over the appropriate code, the number of items needed is inputted, and the order is sent directly to the supplier via computer

Supplies

All supplies received should be examined for damage as well as presence of an accurate packing slip cataloging items shipped.

- If there is any damage or discrepancy, the supplier should be contacted
- A statement with payments due is not enclosed; it is generally sent separately monthly to the practice
- A back order slip may be inserted listing items not immediately available and estimated shipment date
- If any units need to be sent back to the purveyor, they should issue the practice a credit slip indicating there will be no charge for them
- After receipt, the dental assistant should transfer the supplies to a well-organized storage area with older items in front to be utilized first
- In a dental office, certain items will need to be stored in a refrigerator or in a dark, dry spot
- Drugs that are considered controlled substances should be in a locked cabinet

Dental Laboratory Equipment Maintenance

There are many pieces of dental laboratory equipment that may need to be maintained.

- If there is a dental laboratory technician in the office, some maintenance may be done by him or her, but often, it will be the dental assistant's responsibility
- Much of the equipment is related to the taking of impressions, the creation of trays, or the making of casts
- These include the gypsum vibrator, extruder guns, lathes, model trimmer, hydrocolloid conditioning unit, soldering and welding equipment, and vacuum former
- Most of these have explicit manufacturer-provided instructions on their use and maintenance
- There are also spatulas, laboratory knives, reusable impression trays, flexible rubber bowls, and measuring devices that must be cleaned between uses

DENTAL INSTRUMENT CARE

Most dental instruments are made of stainless steel, or occasionally aluminum or high-tech resins.

- They should be cleaned promptly after use by putting them in an ultrasonic bath or instrument washer
- Instruments that cannot be cleaned right away should be put in a presoak temporarily
- Ultrasonic solution should cover all the instruments, which should be separated
- Instruments that have hinges, for example scissors, should be cleaned and later sterilized in the open position
- The instruments are taken out of the ultrasonic bath, held under running water, dried, and then sterilized
- Sterilization techniques (discussed further in the Infection Control Examination) include liquid chemical disinfectants, ethylene oxide, hot glass bead, dry heat, chemical vapor, and steam autoclave sterilization
- The instruments should be dried prior to storage
- Some instruments have different or additional maintenance requirements
- For example, burs and handpieces need to be scrubbed first, and since handpieces are attached to a power source via tubing, they need initial flushing and lubrication

DANB Practice Test

Want to take this practice test in an online interactive format?
Check out the bonus page, which includes interactive practice questions and
much more: **https://www.mometrix.com/bonus948/danboa**

1. A patient receiving dental radiographs mentions a history of radon exposure at home. What type of radiation is radon classified as?

a. Cosmic radiation
b. Background radiation
c. Terrestrial radiation
d. Medical radiation

2. Between orthodontic treatments, patients should visit their general orthodontist to receive cleanings and other preventive measures including various screenings for cancer. Which one of the following is the muscle found in the neck that is commonly assessed by the orthodontist or dental hygienist during preventive care visits?

a. Hyoglossus
b. Stylohyoid
c. Sternocleidomastoid
d. Internal pterygoid

3. The purpose of collimation is to

a. absorb or block low-energy radiation photons.
b. determine the maximum voltage during exposure.
c. determine the shading and visibility of the image.
d. restrict a radiographic beam to a specific size.

4. A new patient is having an exam prior to undergoing orthodontic treatment and is worried about a piece of tissue that is attaching the upper lip to the gum tissue above the two front teeth. The patient is not sure if it is a normal structure or if it is an anomaly and would like to address it. What is the name of this structure?

a. Mucobuccal fold
b. Labial mandibular tissue
c. Labial frenulum
d. Vestibular fold

5. A patient comes into the dental clinic and has noticeably large and dense bone in the head and neck region compared to a standard dental patient. Which one of the following modifications can be made to the dental machine settings to ensure that the resulting image is acceptable?

a. The milliamperage should be decreased.
b. The kilovoltage peak should be increased.
c. The exposure time should be reduced.
d. The machine will correct itself automatically based on the patient's tissue and bone density.

154

6. What muscle in the mouth helps control the mandible and can also become tired or cramped during long orthodontic appointments during which the patient's mouth has to remain open for extended periods of time?

    a. Masseter
    b. Genioglossus
    c. Digastric
    d. Trapezius

7. When reviewing nutrition with a new orthodontic patient, the orthodontic assistant should advise him or her to limit foods such as sugar, crackers, cookies, candy, and soda. These are all examples of:

    a. complex carbohydrates.
    b. dietary fiber.
    c. simple sugars.
    d. soluble fiber.

8. The orthodontic assistant has draped the patient, donned PPE, and is preparing to apply topical anesthetic gel at the site where local anesthetic will be injected. What should the orthodontic assistant do next?

    a. Review patient's allergies, medications, and experiences with local and/or topical anesthetics.
    b. Rinse patient's mouth.
    c. Dry the area of application.
    d. Apply applicator with gel to the site.

9. Parents present to the orthodontic office with their 7-year-old child after being referred by their primary dentist. The concern is that the child's upper front teeth are starting to stick out more than normal. After a careful examination, the orthodontist indicates that this is a result of tongue thrusting by the child. Which one of the following is the type of tongue thrusting that is causing this condition?

    a. Anterior tongue thrusting
    b. Lateral tongue thrusting
    c. Fan tongue thrusting
    d. Distal tongue thrusting

10. The orthodontist is conducting an examination on a new orthodontic patient and instructs the orthodontic assistant to chart a class V area of decay on tooth #8 that must be restored by the general dentist prior to initiating orthodontic therapy. What should the orthodontic assistant note in this patient's chart?

    a. There is decay on the inside surface of the lower right front tooth.
    b. There is decay on the incisal edge of the lower left front tooth.
    c. There is decay on the outer surface near the gum tissue on the upper right front tooth.
    d. There is decay on the biting surface of the upper left front tooth.

11. The dental team needs to adjust a Hawley retainer that no longer fits a patient. Which one of the following is the appropriate tool to use?

a. Contouring plier
b. Three-pronged plier
c. Posterior plier
d. Bird beak plier

12. After a patient completes braces or other forms of orthodontic treatment, a whitening procedure is often requested. This can cause sensitivity in the patient's teeth due to sensations passing through which one of the following structures?

a. The dentin tube
b. The dentinal fiber
c. The nerve pathway
d. The cementum stimulator

13. When documenting implant devices, which of the following information must be included?

a. Manufacturer, lot and serial numbers, and size
b. Size, type, and lot and serial numbers
c. Manufacturer, size, type, lot and serial numbers, and anatomic placement
d. Manufacturer, size, type, lot and serial numbers, anatomic placement, and patient's gender and age

14. What is the most common treatment for supernumerary teeth?

a. Braces
b. No treatment
c. Removal
d. Capping

15. The orthodontic assistant is preparing the tray for the placement of orthodontic bands. Which one of the following is the cement that is commonly used in this procedure because of its ability to release fluoride and its strength?

a. Composite
b. Glass ionomer
c. Mizzy brand Fleck's zinc phosphate cement
d. Prime and bone

16. The orthodontic assistant is recording chart notations when the dentist states that the patient has class I decay on tooth #3. Where is this decay located?

a. Mesial surface
b. Distal surface
c. Occlusal surface
d. Incisal surface

17. When patients experience the first few days of orthodontic treatment, they often experience some discomfort in the oral cavity. This is most often secondary to the fibers that hold the tooth structure being pulled out of their normal position allowing for tooth movement and bone repositioning. What is the name of the structure that these fibers combine to form?

   a. Periodontal ligament
   b. Interradicular septum
   c. Lining mucosa
   d. Coronal pulp

18. The orthodontic assistant is placing brackets on the enamel surface when the patient asks if the white part of her tooth will come off when the brackets are removed. Which one of the following is an accurate response for the patient?

   a. The white part of the tooth is known as the dentin and has some elasticity to it, allowing for the brackets to shift when needed and will remain intact when the brackets are removed.
   b. The part of the tooth that the brackets are glued to is known as the enamel and is formed to be one of the hardest structures in the body and will not be affected by removal of the brackets.
   c. The cementum is the name of the structure that holds the brackets onto the teeth, and it allows for adhesive fibers to move through the dentin and enamel and adhere to the brackets and will not be affected by their removal.
   d. The brackets are not bonded to the white part of the tooth; they are bonded to the area where the white meets the yellow allowing for a very deep and strong bond to the brackets.

19. When taking a bite registration with silicone material, the material should set up

   a. within seconds.
   b. in 1 minute.
   c. in 2 minutes.
   d. in 4 minutes.

20. The orthodontist is installing new radiology equipment and has purchased a machine that will produce x-rays using a kilovolt peak setting of 70. What is the required size of the aluminum filtration component that must be used in combination with this machine to allow for proper filtration?

   a. 1.5 mm thick
   b. 2 mm thick
   c. 2.5 mm thick
   d. 3 mm thick

21. Which one of the following is NOT a component of an effective instrument transfer during an orthodontic procedure?

   a. Anticipation by the orthodontic assistant
   b. Understanding of the instrument sequence
   c. Knowledge of which hand to use with a right- or left-handed orthodontist
   d. Understanding how to use class IV motions during transfers

22. An 11-year-old patient presents at the orthodontic office for a consultation visit. She is currently in the mixed dentition stage with the only remaining primary tooth remaining being the lower right second molar. Using the universal numbering system, what is the correct name for this remaining primary second molar?

a. Tooth A
b. Tooth J
c. Tooth K
d. Tooth T

23. A patient is having her braces (brackets, wires, elastic bands, and molar bands) removed. What is the correct initial procedure?

a. Remove the brackets.
b. Remove the elastic bands.
c. Remove the molar bands.
d. Provide local anesthetic.

24. When considering the type of arch wire to use, the orthodontist desires one that is very flexible and appropriate for the beginning phase of the orthodontic treatment, especially for movement of the anterior teeth. Which one of the following would meet those criteria?

a. Optiflex
b. Nickel titanium
c. Stainless steel
d. Beta titanium

25. A patient presents for an initial orthodontic consultation and states that he would like to change his bite. Currently his upper front teeth are behind the bottom front teeth, and he would like to reverse that so that his upper front teeth are in front of his lower front teeth. What classification of malocclusion does he want to correct?

a. Class I
b. Class II, division 1
c. Class II, division 2
d. Class III

26. When the orthodontic assistant is reviewing the patient's clinical record, which one of the following should NOT be found in that record?

a. The insurance provider
b. The sequence of past appointments
c. Treatment plans
d. Dental radiographs

27. MRI would be most effective for

a. diagnosis of disease of the salivary glands.
b. diagnosis of facial fracture.
c. evaluation of orthodontic prosthesis.
d. evaluation of malocclusion.

28. One important role of an orthodontic assistant is to ligate the arch wire. What is the purpose of ligating the arch wire?

    a. To bend the arch wire for placement
    b. To remove any cement from the arch wire
    c. To hold the arch wire in place
    d. To prepare the arch wire for removal

29. The orthodontist has asked the orthodontic assistant to capture an image that will give more information about the patient's facial anatomy as well as the projected growth patterns that need to be accounted for prior to orthodontic therapy. Which one of the following types of images will show this information?

    a. Posteroanterior
    b. Lateral cephalometric
    c. Temporomandibular
    d. Panoramic

30. What is the first step when using light-cure adhesives with phosphoric acid etchant to bond brackets to a tooth?

    a. Dry tooth.
    b. Polish tooth with pumice.
    c. Cover tooth surface with etchant.
    d. Place cheek retractors.

31. The orthodontic assistant is conducting an exam on a new patient prior to the orthodontist coming into the operatory. The patient mentions noticing a white line on the roof of the mouth and asks the orthodontic assistant what that is. The orthodontic assistant knows that this line is referred to as what?

    a. Tuberosity
    b. Mental protuberance
    c. Medial palatal suture
    d. Lacrimal bone

32. The orthodontic assistant is setting up before starting a treatment to place separators in a patient and realizes that the standard plastic separators commonly used for this procedure are out of stock. Which one of the following is an acceptable alternative?

    a. Steel separating springs
    b. Composite embrasure brackets
    c. Avoiding the separators and moving forward to orthodontic bands
    d. Resin interproximal spacers

33. When considering the development of radiation protection mechanisms, it is important to understand which tissues of the body have high and low sensitivity to radiation. Of the following tissues, which one has the lowest sensitivity to ionizing radiation?

    a. Bone marrow
    b. Connective tissue
    c. Oral mucosa
    d. Nerve tissue

34. What does it mean when the orthodontic assistant must perform functions under direct supervision?

  a. The orthodontist must be physically present in the orthodontic office when the procedure is performed.
  b. The orthodontist must be aware of the procedure but does not need to be physically present in the office.
  c. The orthodontist does not need to authorize the procedure but must be present in the office when it is performed.
  d. The orthodontist must be next to the orthodontic assistant and must watch the procedure from beginning to end.

35. When assisting during an orthodontic procedure, if the orthodontist is right-handed and positioned in the operator's activity zone at approximately the 9 to 12 o'clock position (patient's head at 12 o'clock), where is the assistant positioned?

  a. 12 to 2 o'clock
  b. 2 to 4 o'clock
  c. 4 to 6 o'clock
  d. 7 to 9 o'clock

36. Dental nutrition is an important aspect of preventive care. Which one of the following is a category of food that directly leads to the formation of decay and should be discussed with the patient as part of a nutrition program?

  a. High-density foods
  b. Cariogenic foods
  c. Polyunsaturated fats
  d. Triglycerides

37. It is common practice in orthodontics to remove premolar teeth when there is crowding in order to free up additional space. What function is lost when the premolar teeth are removed?

  a. The ability to cut into food with minimal effort
  b. The ability to tear into food using force
  c. The ability to hold and grind food
  d. The ability to chew and grind food

38. An orthodontist is in the middle of a complex procedure involving full-mouth braces. Due to the difficulty of the case, the orthodontist has decided that she no longer wishes to provide services to the patient and tells the staff to discontinue any scheduled appointments for that patient or her family. The orthodontist advises staff to simply say that the schedules are full and the patient should look for another orthodontist in the area. This is an example of:

  a. malpractice.
  b. res gestae.
  c. implied consent.
  d. abandonment.

39. When measuring the patient's blood pressure, the orthodontic assistant records a systolic reading of 128 mmHg and a diastolic reading of 79 mmHg. Which blood pressure category would these measurements fall into?

a. Normal blood pressure
b. Prehypertension
c. Hypertension stage 1
d. Hypertension stage 2

40. The orthodontist is preparing to place bands on a new patient who has just had separators removed. Which one of the following is the correct way for the orthodontist to place the bands on to ensure placement at the desired location without any improper bending or manipulation?

a. Apply pressure on the facial surface of the band.
b. Apply pressure on the buccal and lingual surfaces of the band.
c. Apply pressure on the mesial and distal surfaces of the band.
d. Apply pressure on the occlusal surface of the band.

41. Which type of wax is appropriate for an orthodontic patient who complains of pain and irritation from brackets?

a. Boxing wax
b. Sticky wax
c. Utility wax
d. Undercut wax

42. During an exam, a patient is describing to the orthodontic assistant that the outside of the upper front teeth feels rough. The orthodontic assistant identifies that there is leftover cement (which can be removed) from the bonding on the brackets. When the orthodontic assistant informs the orthodontist, what surface of the teeth should be reported as having the cement?

a. Lingual surface
b. Distal surface
c. Facial surface
d. Mesial surface

43. The correct method of inserting a tray for an impression and seating it is to insert the tray

a. straight into the mouth and press onto the teeth from front to back.
b. straight into the mouth and press onto the teeth from back to front.
c. sideways into the mouth, rotate, and press onto the teeth from back to front.
d. sideways into the mouth, rotate, and press onto the teeth from front to back.

44. The orthodontic assistant is preparing to take digital bitewings when the patient with a background in radiology asks about the type of the wavelength that is used in dental imaging. Which one of the following is the correct response?

a. Short wavelengths with high velocity
b. Long wavelengths with low velocity
c. Short wavelengths with low velocity
d. Long wavelengths with high velocity

45. A fully credentialed orthodontist must provide all patients with a basic, acceptable level of care. This level of care is determined by what is being provided by other orthodontists in similar demographics and of similar status against specific identifiable standards. This is an example of:

    a. direct supervision.
    b. expressed contract.
    c. standard of care.
    d. reciprocity.

46. When instructing a patient about wearing sequential plastic aligners, the orthodontic assistant should advise the patient to

    a. wear the aligners at all times.
    b. remove to brush and floss the teeth and while eating.
    c. remove to brush and floss the teeth only.
    d. wear during the day but remove at night.

47. During an appointment in which the orthodontist is placing molar bands, which instrument should the orthodontic assistant have ready?

    a. Pin and ligature stick
    b. Posterior band stick
    c. Three-pronged pliers
    d. Bite stick

48. At which age should the upper permanent incisors appear in the oral cavity?

    a. 6–8 years
    b. 7–9 years
    c. 9–11 years
    d. 11–12 years

49. Which one of the following is a procedure in which the orthodontic assistant must use a fulcrum action?

    a. Taking dental radiographs
    b. Placing orthodontic separators
    c. Placing cement onto dental brackets
    d. Providing the patient with a limited rinse

50. Which pliers are used to place and remove archwires?

    a. Prong
    b. Edgewise
    c. Howe
    d. Bird beak

51. A patient is receiving a final cleaning at the general dentist prior to having bands and brackets placed by the orthodontist. The dentist asks the dental assistant to capture images that will allow viewing of any decay that may be hidden once the bands and brackets are placed. What type of images should the dental assistant take?

    a. Bitewing images
    b. Occlusal images
    c. Periapical images
    d. Vertical phosphor storage plates

52. The orthodontic assistant is conducting a medical/dental history and the adult patient states that she takes 8 medications for asthma and "a heart condition," but she does not know the names of the drugs and cannot be more specific. What should the orthodontic assistant do?

    a. Note in the chart the number and purpose of the drugs.
    b. Ask the patient if she knows if she is taking a "blood thinner."
    c. Set an appointment for the patient to return at another time when she can bring the names of the medications with her.
    d. Notify the orthodontist that the patient may be at risk.

53. A coolant is used with a high-speed dental handpiece to prevent

    a. overheating of the unit.
    b. pulpal damage.
    c. too rapid cutting.
    d. burning of the mouth.

54. The orthodontic assistant has just seated the patient in the correct position to work on braces on the lower teeth. When the assistant seats themselves, what is the correct distance that should be placed between the orthodontic assistant's face and the patient's face in order to reduce ergonomic strain?

    a. 8–10 inches apart
    b. 10–12 inches apart
    c. 12–14 inches apart
    d. 14–16 inches apart

55. All staff in the dental office must follow the protocols set forth in the HIPAA standards. What does HIPAA stand for?

    a. Health Information Protection and Accessibility Act
    b. Health Insurance Portability and Accountability Act
    c. Health Informatics Planning and Accountability Act
    d. Health Information Programming and Accessibility Act

56. Which one of the following is the correct dental tool that is used after the ligature wire to remove any loose ends?

    a. Ligature tying pliers
    b. Weingart scissors
    c. Posterior ligature cutter
    d. Pin and ligature cutter

57. When preparing pastes for a polysulfide impression, in what order should the pastes be mixed?

    a. First the syringe material and then the tray material
    b. First the tray material and then the syringe material
    c. Both materials at the same time
    d. Any order

58. When the dental team uses wire ligature ties, what is the appropriate length that can be left at the end of the ligature tie after it is wrapped around the bracket?

    a. 1–2 mm
    b. 2–3 mm
    c. 3–5 mm
    d. 4–5 mm

59. During conversation with a new patient, the orthodontic assistant learns that this patient was employed at a nuclear power plant that was found to have a radiation leak to which the patient was exposed. An investigation revealed that because of this radiation leak, many of the employees developed cancer as they aged. What is the term that is used to describe the time from the exposure at the power plant to the development of cancer later in the patient's life?

    a. Dose accumulated rate
    b. Genetic effect period
    c. Somatic accumulation effect
    d. Latent period

60. In the Universal tooth numbering system for adults, how are the upper central incisors numbered (right to left)?

    a. 2 and 1
    b. E and F
    c. 8 and 9
    d. 11 and 21

61. The orthodontic assistant is performing a polish on a patient with a pumice mixture prior to placing dental brackets. Which classification of movement would be used for this procedure?

    a. Class I
    b. Class II
    c. Class III
    d. Class IV

62. Which one of the following is commonly used in orthodontics to move the upper first molar toward the back of the mouth to allow for additional room to be created in the arch?

    a. Traction device
    b. Hawley retainer
    c. Retention retainer
    d. Face bow

63. Which one of the following is the next step after any orthodontic therapy to maintain the new positioning of the teeth?

   a. Retention
   b. Positioning
   c. Reevaluation
   d. Cement removal

64. During orthodontic treatment, the patient's biting and chewing movements will be altered by the force of the brackets and arch wire. Which one of the following is the name given to these types of biting and chewing movements?

   a. Malocclusion
   b. Centric occlusion
   c. Functional occlusion
   d. Distoclusion

65. The orthodontic assistant is charting the treatment that needs to be done as well as what restorations currently exist in a new patient's mouth. Which color should the orthodontic assistant use to chart the restorations that need to be completed?

   a. Blue
   b. Black
   c. Green
   d. Red

66. When instructing patients in the proper flossing techniques, the orthodontic assistant should advise patient to keep the working length of the floss at about

   a. 1.0–1.5 inches.
   b. 3–5 inches.
   c. 2–4 inches.
   d. 1.5–3.0 inches.

67. Which of the following radiographic procedures is the best choice for diagnosing an abscessed tooth?

   a. Periapical radiograph
   b. Occlusal film
   c. Bitewing radiograph
   d. Posteroanterior extraoral radiograph

68. During the placement of the initial orthodontic bands and brackets, the orthodontic assistant notices an extra area of enamel on the inside of the patient's first upper molar. The assistant then looks at the opposite side of the mouth and notices that same structure on the opposite molar. The assistant is concerned that this possible abnormality could affect the placement of the orthodontic bands. In discussing this with the orthodontist, the orthodontist identifies this as a normal structure called the:

   a. cingulum.
   b. lingual ridge.
   c. fossa.
   d. cusp of Carabelli.

69. The orthodontic assistant is preparing to measure the patient's heart rate and would like to use the radial artery for this measurement. Which one of the following is the correct area for the orthodontic assistant to measure the heart rate?

    a. Just above the temple on the side of the forehead
    b. Inner surface of the forearm, on the side of the pinky finger
    c. Inner surface of the wrist, on the side of the thumb
    d. Alongside the larynx

70. The orthodontist is reviewing a set of bitewing images taken on an orthodontic patient to evaluate for interproximal decay. The orthodontist states that the images are slightly distorted with blurriness throughout the images. Which one of the following is the term given to the blurriness that the orthodontist is referring to?

    a. Density
    b. Contrast
    c. Penumbra
    d. Magnification

71. When fitting and cementing bands onto the molars, which one of the following is correct?

    a. The teeth need to be dried off and protected against moisture prior to mixing the dental cement and placing the bands.
    b. The band should be held by the outside surfaces with the surface that will go toward the gum tissue facing downward.
    c. After the band is placed on the tooth, the orthodontic assistant must transfer the band pusher to the orthodontist for use to seat the band on the tooth.
    d. The patient must avoid biting down on the band once it is seated to prevent trauma to the gum tissue.

72. When preparing the bands that will be used in an appointment, the orthodontist asks the assistant to apply the round tubes that are commonly used to the bands that will be placed on the first molars during the procedure. What is the name of these round tubes?

    a. Lingual arch tubes
    b. Labial tubes
    c. Edgewise tubes
    d. Headgear tubes

73. The orthodontic assistant is reviewing the treatment plan with the patient. All treatment options and costs must be reviewed with the patient regardless of what the orthodontist thinks is best. This is an example of which ethical principle?

    a. Autonomy
    b. Beneficence
    c. Justice
    d. Veracity

74. Which one of the following is an important aspect of preventive dentistry and oral health education and serves as a way to close off small crevices in the biting surfaces of teeth?

    a. Dental caries
    b. Composite fillings
    c. Fluoride treatment
    d. Dental sealants

75. The orthodontic assistant is preparing to press the exposure button on a panoramic image. Which one of the following is a correct description that can be given to the patient regarding what will happen once the exposure button is pressed?

a. The panoramic machine tubehead will rotate behind the patient's head, while any digital plates will rotate in front of the patient's head.
b. The x-ray beam will emit from the tubehead measuring a 2.75-inch circumference when it penetrates the patient's skin.
c. The panoramic exposure on the patient will last for 60–80 seconds depending on the density of the patient's tissue.
d. The machine will stop halfway through the exposure, allowing for the patient to be repositioned prior to finishing the exposure.

76. Following the removal of brackets and the completion of orthodontics, the orthodontist may use a high- or slow-speed handpiece to smooth out the enamel surface of the tooth. Care must be taken so as not to remove too much structure from this portion of the tooth; otherwise, it could lead to exposure of which one of the following?

a. The coronal pulp
b. The apical foramen
c. The radicular fibers
d. The dentin

77. The dental team is reviewing a new patient's chart that has been sent over by the patient's general dentist. The orthodontic assistant notices that the patient's wisdom teeth all have been circled in red and asks the orthodontist what this means. What is the correct response?

a. These are teeth that have been identified as missing as a result of extraction, or they were congenitally missing.
b. These are teeth that are not visible in the mouth due to a lack of eruption. They are present and should be noted in the chart, but they have yet to erupt.
c. These teeth are identified as needing to be extracted prior to the orthodontic treatment.
d. Crowns are found on these teeth and should be left out of the orthodontic treatment planning.

78. When should radiographic screening be done prior to conducting a history and physical exam?

a. Never
b. For new patients only
c. For patients who have not been seen in over a year
d. For new patients who report chronic disease

79. Under the guidance of the orthodontist when the office is short-staffed, the orthodontic assistant manipulates the arch wire of a patient during a visit. This is outside of the legal scope of practice for this assistant. What type of law has been violated by the assistant's action?

a. Tort law
b. Civil law
c. Criminal law
d. Contract law

80. The orthodontist is preparing to place the orthodontic bands on a new patient. Which one of the following choices lists the correct teeth where these bands should be placed?

    a. Upper and lower first premolars
    b. Upper and lower first and second premolars
    c. Upper and lower first and second molars
    d. Upper and lower first, second, and third molars

81. What should the orthodontic assistant use when placing elastic separators to prepare for molar bands?

    a. Prong pliers
    b. Hemostat
    c. Edgewise pliers
    d. Separating pliers

82. A patient with type 1 diabetes mellitus becomes increasingly agitated and aggressive and appears disoriented with warm moist skin and rapid pulse. What is the most likely cause?

    a. Hypoglycemia
    b. Anxiety
    c. Hyperglycemia
    d. Anaphylaxis

83. A patient presents to the orthodontic office and, during the examination, it is noted that the patient's upper premolars are found in a lingual position or inside the lower premolars. What is the name given to this type of premolar placement?

    a. Crowding
    b. Distoclusion
    c. Crossbite
    d. Overjet

84. During a procedure when the orthodontist is adjusting and bending the patient's arch wire, the orthodontist asks the assistant for the 110 pliers. Which one of the following is the correct type of pliers that the orthodontic assistant should transfer to the orthodontist?

    a. Howe pliers
    b. Weingart utility pliers
    c. Three-pronged pliers
    d. Posterior band pliers

85. What is a necessary component of informed consent prior to a procedure?

    a. Names of assisting staff members
    b. Beginning and ending times
    c. Risks and benefits of procedure
    d. Facility statistics regarding procedure

86. A 12-year-old patient comes into the orthodontic clinic for early treatment due to severe tooth spacing. This patient still has a number of baby teeth present that will eventually be lost and be replaced by the permanent, adult teeth. How can these permanent teeth be classified?

    a. Mixed dentition teeth
    b. Primary dentition teeth
    c. Succedaneous teeth
    d. Deciduous teeth

87. When placing orthodontic elastomeric separators, what is the most effective technique that will prevent discomfort to the patient and reduce the time needed to perform procedure?

    a. Use a seesaw motion to maneuver the separator between the teeth.
    b. Use a pressure technique, pressing the separator between the teeth with force.
    c. Use the shepherd's hook of the explorer to pull the separator between the teeth.
    d. Have the patient bite down onto the separator to force it into the proximal space between the teeth.

88. A dental team is evaluating a set of radiographs that were submitted by a general dentistry office for a new patient and is concerned because the majority of the upper images are missing the root tips for the back teeth. Which one of the following is the cause of the lack of root tips on the images?

    a. When the images were exposed, the patient moved between when the dental assistant left the room and when the exposure button was pressed.
    b. The side-to-side angle of the dental tubehead was incorrect.
    c. The dental tubehead was not placed correctly over the sensor in the mouth.
    d. The vertical angle of the dental tubehead was incorrect.

89. An orthodontic assistant trained in CPR is present when a 68-year-old patient experiences a cardiac arrest. The assistant calls 9-1-1 and shouts for help. The AED is in another room. What is the correct initial action for the assistant after briefly assessing for consciousness?

    a. Administer chest compressions only at 100/min.
    b. Administer CPR at rate of 30 chest compressions at 100/min, followed by 2 ventilations (30:2).
    c. Obtain the AED and administer shocks prior to starting CPR.
    d. Administer CPR at rate of 20 chest compressions at 60/min, followed by 2 ventilations (20:2).

90. A patient who has HIV/AIDS exhibits painful white cheesy-appearing lesions throughout the mouth with loss of taste. What is the most likely cause?

    a. Candidiasis
    b. Herpetic lesions
    c. Erythema multiforme
    d. Pemphigus

91. The orthodontic assistant is asked to chart the fact that teeth #1, #16, and #17 are impacted. Which one of the following is the correct charting notation to use for these three teeth?

a. Cross out the teeth with a blue X.
b. Circle the teeth in red.
c. Color the teeth in blue.
d. Circle the roots of the teeth in red.

92. A patient who recently finished wearing braces is asking the orthodontic team which toothpaste can be used to help whiten the teeth. The orthodontic team should recommend toothpaste with which one of the following active ingredients?

a. Sodium fluoride
b. Triclosan
c. Potassium nitrate
d. Hydrogen peroxide

93. The orthodontic assistant is preparing a patient for a new three-dimensional image that will be taking place at the orthodontic office that will have the ability to show structures and images in three dimensions. Which one of the following is the name of that image?

a. Periapical
b. Panoramic
c. Bitewing
d. Cone beam computed tomography

94. In dentistry, there are certain organs of the body that have been identified as critical organs. These areas are highly sensitive to radiation and should avoid exposure when possible. Which one of the following is an example of a critical organ?

a. Salivary gland
b. Thyroid gland
c. Kidney
d. Developing bone

95. A 32-year-old patient presents for a check-in visit for an orthodontic treatment. The orthodontist indicates to the assistant that the band on tooth #30 is loose and needs to be recemented onto the tooth. Which quadrant is this tooth found in?

a. Upper right
b. Lower right
c. Upper left
d. Lower left

96. The orthodontic assistant is setting up for a quick appointment to remove elastomeric rings that were placed during a previous appointment to prepare the teeth for orthodontic bands. Which one of the following is an instrument that would be appropriate to include in the tray setup?

a. Orthodontic scaler
b. Bird beak pliers
c. Band plugger
d. Ligature director

97. The orthodontic assistant received notification that her national certification was expiring and neglected to pay the renewal fee. This resulted in a lapse of her certification, something that is required in her state of employment. This is an example of a(n):

   a. infraction.
   b. misdemeanor.
   c. ethical dilemma.
   d. dental felony.

98. Which one of the following structures holds the arch wire in place on each tooth?

   a. Bracket
   b. Band
   c. Resin
   d. Ligature

99. Tensing of which of the following muscles of mastication is associated with temporomandibular joint (TMJ) syndrome?

   a. Masseter
   b. Temporalis
   c. Medial pterygoid
   d. Lateral pterygoid

100. When planning out a sequence of orthodontic appointments, which one of the following is correct?

   a. Separator placement, band placement, arch wire, bonding of brackets, adjustment checks
   b. Arch wire, band placement, separator placement, bonding of brackets, adjustment checks
   c. Separator placement, band placement, bonding of brackets, arch wire, adjustment checks
   d. Band placement, separator placement, bonding of brackets, arch wire, adjustment checks

101. An important part of a healthy mouth is the salivary flow rate. Which one of the following is a main function of saliva and an important reason to monitor the salivary flow?

   a. To help clear food particles in the oral cavity during and after chewing
   b. To reduce the harmful minerals that are present on the teeth in the linea alba
   c. To introduce healthy bacteria to fight off decay
   d. To serve as a direct source of vitamin A that allows the teeth to remineralize

102. Which one of the following is an acrylic, removable retention device created following a patient's orthodontic treatment?

   a. Composite retainer
   b. Hawley retainer
   c. Ligature retainer
   d. Weingart retainer

103. Which one of the following is the correct action that the orthodontic team should take to ensure a positive patient visit?

    a. Ensure that disinfected dental instruments are available for use.

    b. Review the patient's medical and dental records prior to the patient's appointment.

    c. Avoid collecting payment and insurance information until the patient is present in the office.

    d. Make sure that the treatment room is free of any trays or dental instruments already setup for use.

104. The best method to use when examining the dorsum of the tongue is to ask the patient to

    a. push the tongue toward the right or left cheek.

    b. protrude the tongue.

    c. lift the tongue toward the hard palate.

    d. place the tip of the tongue against the back of the lower teeth.

105. The amount of radiation that a patient is exposed to can be measured in roentgens using the traditional units of measuring radiation. What is the equivalent to the roentgen when using the International System of Units measuring system?

    a. Gray

    b. Sievert

    c. Coulomb per kilogram

    d. Rad

106. Which type of radiographic imagining is indicated for a patient to evaluate crowding and presence of supernumerary teeth?

    a. Bitewing

    b. Periapical

    c. Occlusal

    d. Panoramic

107. The orthodontic assistant is assisting a right-handed doctor in the placement of bands and brackets for braces. Using the clock concept, which one of the following is the correct time zone in which the transfer of instruments should occur?

    a. The 7–12 o'clock position

    b. The 5–8 o'clock position

    c. The 6–10 o'clock position

    d. The 3–7 o'clock position

108. When setting up a treatment tray, the armamentarium should be placed according to

    a. sequence of use, starting from the left and going to the right.

    b. sequence of use, starting from the right and going to the left.

    c. size, with the largest on the far right and smallest on the far left.

    d. size, with the largest on the far left and the smallest on the far right.

109. Which of the following is the term used to describe one developing tooth that partially divides into two teeth?

a. Fusion
b. Gemination
c. Dens invaginatus
d. Concrescence

110. Which one of the following is a correct statement pertaining to the lingual retainer?

a. It is a removeable retainer commonly used following orthodontic therapy.
b. It is placed from the first premolar on one side to the first premolar on the other side.
c. It is only placed on the upper arch.
d. It is made of light steel wire.

111. The orthodontic assistant is preparing a patient for a panoramic image exposure. The orthodontic assistant asks the patient to bite into a notch located in the area where the patient's teeth are placed and states that the notch helps ensure that the teeth are in the imaging layer where the machine assumes they are. What is the name of this imaging layer?

a. Cephalostat
b. Frankfort plane
c. Focal trough
d. Digital layer

112. Which one of the following is a sugar substitute that the orthodontic team can inform the patient of that serves to decrease the risk of dental decay during orthodontic treatment?

a. Xylitol
b. Aspartame
c. Truvia
d. Saccharin

113. Which one of the following is an important step that must occur before the dental team can cement on the brackets used for braces?

a. The teeth must be polished with an extra-fine sandpaper disk.
b. The patient must be given a fluoride treatment to prepare the dentin tubules.
c. The teeth must be cleaned with pumice using a prophy cup.
d. The patient must brush the teeth for a minimum of 1 minute.

114. Which one of the following is a newer option available in orthodontics that allows for the patient to eliminate the need of metal braces but has the ability to provide the same effects?

a. Hawley retainer
b. Vacuum-formed clear aligner
c. Elastics
d. Overbraces

115. In the Palmer tooth notation system for deciduous teeth, what does the following notation refer to?

⌐A

a. Upper left central incisor
b. Upper right central incisor
c. Lower left central incisor
d. Lower right central incisor

116. The dental team must follow safety precautions when exposing patients to ionizing radiation in order to prevent small exposures over a prolonged period of time. Which one of the following can be used to describe those small amounts of radiation exposure?

a. Acute radiation exposure
b. Chronic radiation exposure
c. Cumulative radiation exposure
d. Somatic radiation exposure

117. A 10-year-old patient presents in the orthodontic office for a consultation. The caregiver is wondering when the patient will get the second set of adult teeth in the back of the mouth on top. The dental team determines that the caregiver is referring to the patient's second molars. What is the best answer regarding when these teeth will erupt into the oral cavity?

a. 10–11 years of age
b. 12–13 years of age
c. 13–years of age
d. 14–15 years of age

118. A patient presents for an orthodontic examination after having jogged there. Which one of the following would the dental team expect to note in the patient's check-in exam?

a. Decreased respiratory rate
b. Increased blood pressure
c. Decreased heart rate
d. Hypoxia

119. When the orthodontic assistant is positioning themselves for a patient visit, which one of the following should be avoided?

a. Placing the feet flat on the floor
b. Being seated as far back on the operator's chair as possible
c. Positioning the thighs so that they are perpendicular to the floor with the knees higher than the hips
d. Positioning the backrest so it is supporting the lower back

120. A new orthodontic assistant has just joined the team. He notices that the other staff in the office are often talking down to other staff members and patients. What basic ethical principle is the new assistant demonstrating by NOT engaging with or participating in the negative talk about other staff and patients?

a. Nonmaleficence
b. Veracity
c. Autonomy
d. Confidentiality

121. The Council on Radiation Protection and Measurements developed limits that occupationally exposed workers must adhere to when accounting for radiation exposure. What are the limits for dental workers?

    a. 5 rem per year
    b. 6 rem per year
    c. 7 rem per year
    d. 8 rem per year

122. The orthodontic assistant is transferring hinged posterior band removal pliers to the orthodontist. Which one of the following is the correct action for this type of transfer?

    a. The pliers should be transferred so that the handle portion of the pliers is placed into the orthodontist's palm.
    b. The pliers should be transferred in the open position.
    c. A two-handed instrument transfer technique should be avoided with these pliers.
    d. Due to the weight of the pliers, the orthodontist will pick them up directly from the instrument tray setup.

123. When counseling a parent about dietary intake of non-milk extrinsic sugars to prevent caries in a child, the orthodontic assistant should recommend that non-milk extrinsic sugars be

    a. completely eliminated.
    b. consumed only at mealtimes.
    c. restricted to 5–6 servings per day.
    d. consumed rather than intrinsic sugars.

124. The orthodontic assistant is preparing a patient for an initial consultation. The patient presents with a bite that results in the top teeth completely covering the bottom front teeth when the patient bites them together. What is the name of this type of bite?

    a. Overbite
    b. Overlap
    c. Overjet
    d. Class 1 occlusion

125. When considering the use of stainless-steel ligature ties, which one of the following is accurate?

    a. They are made of 0.015-inch stainless steel material.
    b. They must be placed onto each bracket on each tooth.
    c. The orthodontic assistant always starts from the back of the mouth moving to the front.
    d. They are placed with posterior band pliers.

126. An orthodontic assistant has just started at a new clinic. When starting to chart the oral structures, he notices that the dentist is referring to the teeth by the numbers 1–32. Which numbering system is the dentist using?

    a. International Organization for Standardization system
    b. FDI World Dental Federation (Fédération Dentaire Internationale) notation system
    c. Palmer notation system
    d. Universal numbering system

127. During the production of radiation, heat is generated within the dental tubehead. In order to prevent the tubehead from becoming hot to the touch, which one of the following is found inside the tubehead that has the function to maintain its temperature within?

    a. X-ray tube
    b. Insulating oil
    c. Transformer
    d. Metal housing

128. When a patient is undergoing orthodontic care, it is important for the patient to visit his or her primary dentist to receive fluoride treatments in the form of varnish, gel, or rinses. These types of fluoride treatments are known as:

    a. systemic fluoride.
    b. topical fluoride.
    c. ingestible fluoride.
    d. preventable fluoride.

129. When the arch wire is being placed, which one of the following must occur?

    a. The mark at the center of the arch wire must be lined up between teeth #8 and #9.
    b. The arch wire must be placed in the lingual tubes of the bands.
    c. The ends of the arch wire must stick out through the lingual tubes to ensure they remain in place.
    d. The arch wires should be measured after they are placed in the patient's oral cavity.

130. When setting up the orthodontist's and the assistant's stools in a treatment room, where should the assistant's stool should be positioned?

    a. At the same height as the orthodontist's chair
    b. As far as possible from the patient's side
    c. 1–2 inches below the height of the orthodontist's chair
    d. 4–6 inches above the height of the orthodontist's chair

131. When preparing a patient for a blood pressure measurement, which one of the following is the correct positioning?

    a. Patient lying flat, ankles crossed
    b. Patient's maxillary arch perpendicular to the floor, with the arms folded across the chest
    c. Patient sitting in an upright position, with the legs uncrossed
    d. Patient sitting in the Trendelenburg position, with the legs crossed

132. In orthodontics, which one of the following procedures requires written informed consent?

    a. The insertion of a space maintainer
    b. Procedures that take longer than 1 year to complete
    c. Dental impressions for retainers
    d. Cone beam computed tomography scans and panoramic images

133. During an initial exam, the orthodontic assistant is charting the current status of the patient's oral cavity. The assistant is questioning the patient's upper right quadrant because there are nine teeth in that area versus the standard eight teeth per quadrant according to the universal numbering system. Which one of the following conditions is present and causing the source of confusion?

    a. A supernumerary tooth is present.
    b. Gemination has occurred.
    c. Fusion has taken place.
    d. Bifurcation of two teeth has occurred.

134. The orthodontic assistant is preparing a 7-year-old child for an evaluation, but the child is very anxious. Which of the following is the best initial approach?

    a. Promise the child that the procedure will not hurt.
    b. Tell the child he can wiggle his fingers if something hurts.
    c. Tell the caregiver to comfort the child.
    d. Show the child the equipment and how it works.

135. When using no-mix chemical cure adhesive for bonding, the paste must be

    a. placed on both the tooth and the base of the bracket.
    b. placed on the tooth only.
    c. placed on the base of the bracket only.
    d. mixed with the primer and then placed on both the tooth and the base of the bracket.

136. When the orthodontic assistant places elastomeric separators, how long are they left in the patient's mouth?

    a. Up to 5 days
    b. Up to 1 week
    c. Up to 10 days
    d. Up to 2 weeks

137. The orthodontic assistant is speaking with a patient who has been undergoing radiation therapy for oral cancer. The patient is discussing the effects that the radiation therapy has had on her skin, gum tissue, and teeth including the development of red skin, necrotic gum tissue, and the development of dental decay due to the dry mouth caused by radiation. These effects can be classified as which one of the following?

    a. Somatic effects
    b. Latent effects
    c. Genetic effects
    d. Ionization effects

138. The orthodontic assistant is preparing for the next step following the placement of orthodontic bands and the arch wire and would like to use the plastic material that is connected and can go on multiple teeth in a row. Which one of the following is the type of material that the orthodontic assistant is seeking to use?

    a. Elastic chain ties
    b. Plastic circular ties
    c. Composite bands
    d. Amalgam ligature connectors

139. When reviewing oral hygiene home care with an orthodontic patient, the orthodontic assistant is reviewing how to floss properly: The floss must go between the teeth into the triangular-shaped space that is covered by gum tissue, and then it must be moved against the teeth, under the gum tissue to remove any particles. What is the name of the triangular space that the orthodontic assistant is referring to?

    a. Embrasure
    b. Contact area
    c. Lingual space
    d. Apical triangle

140. As the orthodontic assistant prepares the patient for exposure to bitewing images, the patient asks why the orthodontic assistant stands outside the room because "dental radiation is not harmful." Which one of the following is the correct response?

    a. Any amount of radiation can be harmful; standing outside the room allows for any stray x-ray beams to dissipate before they contact the dental staff.
    b. Dental radiation is safe; it is simply the dental equipment manufacturer's requirement that the dental staff using the machines stand outside of the direct treatment room where exposure takes place.
    c. Dental radiation is comparable to medical radiation and is considered safe for dental team members as long as they are wearing a lead apron. The decision to wear a lead apron during occupational exposure is at the discretion of each orthodontic assistant.
    d. Dental radiation is minimal, but it is still harmful. Standing outside the room is an optional personal safety decision that each staff member can make.

Answer Key and Explanations

1. C: Radon is classified as terrestrial radiation. It is an invisible gas that can be found in many dwellings that have underground or partially underground basements. Certain areas in the United States are found to have higher natural levels of radon compared to others. Exposure to radon can be harmful because it contains ionizing particles that can damage tissue and lead to conditions such as lung cancer. Cosmic radiation is a type of background radiation that comes from outer space and is a type that we are all exposed to throughout daily life.

2. C: The muscle in the neck that is often assessed in screening measures during a routine visit is the sternocleidomastoid—a very large muscle that can be evaluated by having the patient turn the head in various directions and feeling for deficiencies or abnormalities. The neck region is included in the cancer screening at the dental office because it is tied to the oral cavity, head, and neck region and can be overlooked by the general medical community during screenings. The hyoglossus, stylohyoid, and internal pterygoid are other muscles found in other parts of the head and neck region that are not generally part of the standard orthodontic screening evaluation.

3. D: The purpose of collimation is to restrict a radiographic beam to a specific size to reduce the patient's exposure to radiation. The FDA now recommends rectangular collimation instead of round, with the beam not to exceed the size of receptor by more than 2% of the source-to-image receptor distance. This collimation should be routinely used for periapical radiographs and is also recommended for bitewing radiographs. Rectangular collimation reduces radiation exposure and improves image clarity by reducing scatter radiation.

4. C: The name of this structure is the labial frenulum. It is a small piece of tissue that connects the upper lip to the gum tissue and is a normal structure. The mucobuccal and vestibular folds are located in the upper and lower portions of the mouth and are found between the lip and the gum tissue, while the labial mandibular gingiva can be found in the lower portion of the mouth.

5. B: When a patient presents with excess hard or soft tissue, the orthodontic assistant can increase the kilovoltage peak, which will increase the speed at which the x-rays exit the tubehead and interact with the patient. When x-rays are moving at a faster speed, they will have the ability to pass through the additional bone or soft tissue and produce an acceptable and diagnosable image. If this adjustment did not occur, the resulting image would appear light in color, which could result in the orthodontist missing an existing anomaly. The milliamperage and exposure time can also be increased to compensate for a patient with excess hard or soft tissue. This will allow for more x-rays to be generated and expose the patient for a longer period of time.

6. A: The masseter muscle is found in the head and neck area and helps control the lower jaw when the patient holds the jaw open for extended periods of time. This can often lead to discomfort when the muscle starts to cramp. The genioglossus, digastric, and trapezius are other muscles of the head and neck that serve functions outside of the opening or closing of the mouth including movement of the tongue, shoulder blades, and hyoid bone.

7. C: Foods such as sugar, crackers, cookies, candy, and soda are known as simple sugars. These types of foods break down easily in the mouth and should be limited in orthodontic treatment because of their ability to cause weakening of the enamel and decay when consumed and not properly or promptly removed from the teeth. The remnants and bacteria left from these foods can get under the wire and around the brackets that are used in traditional braces, becoming trapped in these hard-to-brush areas, which provides a desirable atmosphere for decalcification.

179

8. A: Prior to applying topical anesthetic, the orthodontic assistant should review the patient's allergies, medications (especially any recent changes), and prior experiences with local and/or topical anesthetics. Then, the patient's mouth is rinsed and the site dried with a gauze pad. The gel is applied to an applicator and the tip of the applicator is placed against the site and left in place until removed for the injection. If numbing is inadequate, a second applicator should be prepared and applied.

9. A: This type of anterior teeth movement is caused by anterior tongue thrusting that occurs when the child and is pushing out on the front teeth from the inside with the tongue. This consistent pressure causes the front teeth to start to move, resulting in overjet, or teeth that stick out. This can be remediated by orthodontic treatment, but interceptive measures must also be included to prevent the child from continuing the anterior tongue thrusting.

10. C: The orthodontic assistant should note in the patient's chart that there is decay on the outer surface near the gum tissue on the upper right front tooth. This tooth is identified as tooth #8 in the universal numbering system. Class V decay is that found on the outer surfaces of any tooth. Decay in any area of the mouth should be restored prior to orthodontic treatment. If it is not, there is the risk of a bracket or band being placed over the decayed area, causing further damage and weakness of the tooth. Regular preventive exams should be maintained as well by patients to ensure the integrity of their oral health throughout orthodontic therapy.

11. D: The bird beak plier is the correct tool for making adjustments to oral appliances including the Hawley retainer. The dental team can place the retainer in the patient's mouth and identify the areas that are not fitting correctly and adjust those areas. The bird beak plier has fine ends that allow for the dental team to manipulate the small metal areas of the Hawley retainer. This is important for maintaining the positioning of the teeth that has been accomplished by the orthodontic treatment that occurred prior to the use of the Hawley retainer.

12. B: Each tooth has a number of structures that form as the tooth forms. The structure that provides sensation to the tooth is called the dentinal fiber. When a patient whitens the teeth, this fiber or nerve can be exposed to the whitening product, which can cause tooth sensitivity. The dental office can help the patient manage by using products that can block the transmission of negative sensitivity by the dentinal fibers.

13. C: Documentation for implants must include manufacturer, size, type, lot and serial number, and anatomic placement. Information should be documented in the patient's permanent record, operative record, and the implant registry. Implants should be stored by manufacturer, type of implant, and size and individually wrapped except for plates and screws that are used together as a unit, and the label should be double-checked before opening on the surgical field to prevent wastage. Implants should never be reused, and bending or modifying should be avoided if possible.

14. C: The most common treatment for supernumerary teeth is removal because the extra teeth may displace or impact adjacent teeth so that permanent teeth may not erupt at all. The supernumerary teeth must usually be removed if the teeth are to align properly. Supernumerary teeth can occur with both deciduous and permanent teeth but are more common in males than females. The teeth are classified as conical (usually in front teeth only) odontoma, supplemental (duplications), and tuberculate.

15. B: Glass ionomer is commonly selected as the type of cement to use when placing bands on the molar teeth. One of the desirable properties of glass ionomers is their ability to release fluoride throughout the time that they are in the mouth. This is important because fluoride can help prevent cavities throughout the orthodontic application when the bands and brackets remain in the mouth. If there are any bacteria under the glass ionomer and band, the fluoride will work to fight them off. Glass ionomers are also very strong and will prevent the bands from coming off throughout the treatment.

16. C: Class I decay is decay that is found on the occlusal surface—in this case, of tooth #3. This is a common location for decay in the posterior teeth because they have deep grooves and crevices where bacteria and food debris can get stuck and missed by brushing and flossing. Another system used to indicate the location of caries or restorations throughout the mouth is Black's cavity classification system, which is very commonly used in clinical charting and assessment.

17. A: The fibers that are found in each tooth socket and help to hold the tooth in place are collectively called the periodontal ligament. These fibers line the tooth socket and attach to the cementum of the tooth and the lamina dura of the socket to serve as a cushion and as an attachment point to hold the tooth in place. When a patient is in the first few days of orthodontic treatment or has just gone in for an adjustment, the teeth are putting pressure in a certain direction on these fibers causing discomfort for many patients. This is allowing for tooth movement in the direction indicated by the orthodontist and is a healthy, normal part of orthodontic treatment.

18. B: Brackets that are glued or bonded to a patient's teeth are attached to the part of the tooth called the enamel, which is the white part of the tooth that the patient is worried will come off. The enamel is one of the hardest and strongest tissues in the body and will not be affected by the placement or removal of the brackets. The brackets are bonded to the enamel to allow the brackets and the wire to pull and move the teeth in the direction that is desired by the orthodontist. The cementum, dentin, and root are all other parts of the tooth but are covered by gum tissue and are deeper layers of the tooth, which are not directly related to the bonding of brackets.

19. C: Silicone bite registration material should set up in about 2 minutes. The silicone material is applied directly to the occlusal surface of the lower teeth with an application gun and then the patient occludes the teeth and holds that position without moving until the material sets. If using wax, it must be softened in hot water and placed into the mouth. The patient bites into the material, and the orthodontic assistant contours the soft wax about the teeth, removes the impression, and places it in cold water to harden.

20. C: The aluminum filtration system that must be used with the machine is one that will have filters 2.5 mm thick. This is required for machines that operate with a kilovolt peak speed of 70 or greater. When this type of setting is used, the x-rays are moving at a faster rate of speed and need a thicker filter to remove any of the weak x-rays so that they do not interact with the patient's tissue and cause unnecessary exposure. Filters that are thinner than 2.5 mm will not have the ability to stop the unnecessary x-rays, and filters that are thicker than 2.5 mm will stop the beneficial x-rays that are needed to produce diagnosable images.

21. D: When transferring dental instruments, the orthodontic assistant and the orthodontist should only use motion classifications I, II, and III. Class IV motions should be avoided because too much of the body is being used, resulting in unnecessary movements and potential ergonomic strain. The orthodontic assistant must have a good understanding of not only when the instruments will be needed by the orthodontist, but also in which order they will be used. This will ensure that the assistant provides the orthodontist with the correct instrument at the correct time. The orthodontic assistant must know that a right-handed orthodontist will be using the left hand to transfer instruments and that a left-handed orthodontist will use the right hand for instrument transfer.

22. D: The name for the patient's lower right primary second molar is tooth T. The universal numbering system uses letters to identify the primary teeth and also to distinguish them from the permanent teeth, which are identified by numbers. Both letters and numbers start in the upper right to the upper left and then down from the lower left to the lower right. In the primary dentition, there are five teeth in each of these four areas resulting in the last tooth, the lower right second molar, being tooth T.

23. B: Since elastic bands are applied last, they must be removed first followed by the wires, brackets, and molar bands. Without molar bands, the wire may be left in place and removed in one piece with the brackets. Removing braces is not a painful procedure and should not require a local anesthetic. After the braces are removed, residue from the bonding agent and sometimes plaque may remain on the teeth, so a high-speed dental handpiece is used to clean and polish the teeth.

24. B: Nickel titanium is the arch wire of choice when the orthodontist needs something that is flexible and appropriate for the beginning stages of braces. This type is best when there is lots of movement to be done with the front teeth as well, and it is effective at gently pulling on the front teeth to move them into position. Other types of arch wire have characteristics that can be beneficial for certain treatments including stainless steel and beta titanium being strong and Optiflex being a newer type of wire that does not appear so metallic in the mouth offering the patient more pleasing aesthetics. This type of wire has a glass coating on it and is a good choice for when lighter movement forces are needed.

25. D: Class III malocclusion, also known as mesioclusion, occurs when the upper front teeth are located behind the lower front teeth. Although this is often an aesthetic concern, it can also impact the patient's chewing movements and may be corrected through extensive orthodontic therapy. Other classifications of malocclusion include classes I and II. Class II includes divisions 1 and 2. These classes of occlusion are also common in orthodontic patients and can be corrected to improve patients' aesthetic and functional concerns.

26. A: The insurance provider should not be included in the patent's clinical record. Any finance-related information should not be included in the clinical record because it should contain only information related to the clinical care of the patient. This includes the dental chart and any notations about the dentition and treatment provided. Current and previous treatment plans will also be found in the chart, as well as detailed notes about the patient's history. Any dental images captured will also be part of the clinical chart. It is beneficial to keep these separate to avoid any discrimination or service interruption due to finance-related concerns during patient care.

27. A: The best use of the MRI would be to diagnose disease of the salivary gland. The MRI provides excellent visualization of soft tissues but CT and standard radiographs provide better visualization of hard tissues, so the MRI would not be used to diagnose facial fractures. MRI may be contraindicated if the patient has a metal-containing orthodontic prosthesis. MRI is expensive and time-consuming, so other methods should be used to evaluate a condition, such as malocclusion, when appropriate.

28. C: Ligating the arch wire is a method of ensuring that the wire stays in place throughout the treatment. It is the force from this wire that is placed in each bracket on each tooth that moves the teeth to their desired position. If the arch wire consistently falls off the teeth, the patient would be visiting the orthodontic office almost daily, which would not result in good patient relations nor effective dental treatment. There are several materials that the dental team can use for this process including wire and elastic ties.

29. B: The image that will show the orthodontist the current state of the patient's facial anatomy is the lateral cephalometric image. By viewing where the structures are currently located, the orthodontist can make estimates on how the orthodontic therapy should work and may use this image to determine the exact type of orthodontic therapy to administer to the patient. Posteroanterior, temporomandibular, and panoramic images are all valuable in dentistry, but they do not have the ability to show the facial structures in the views needed to accurately assess a patient's orthodontic needs.

30. B: The first step is to thoroughly polish the surface of the tooth with pumice and then rinse. Cheek retractors are placed and the tooth dried before it is covered with etchant, which is left in place for about 20–30 seconds and then rinsed for about 10 seconds using air and water combination, being careful to suction the solution so that the etchant does not contact tissue. The tooth should be protected from saliva and dried thoroughly and then sealant applied to the tooth and adhesive to the bracket. After application, the adhesive is light cured for 10–40 seconds.

31. C: The white line that the patient and the orthodontic assistant are noticing on the roof of the patient's mouth is called the medial palatal suture. This is the place where the two bones that form the roof of the mouth joined during formation, and the white line indicates the area where the tissue connected and joined together. The tuberosity, mental protuberance, and lacrimal bone are other bones found in the skull that can be identified during a radiographic exam.

32. A: The acceptable alternative for standard orthodontic separators are steel separating springs. The separators and steel separating springs can both be inserted between the teeth and will provide a very small shift in the teeth, allowing for a greater space between the teeth that needs bands to be placed. This is not an aspect of orthodontic therapy that can be avoided because, if this step is not completed, the orthodontist may not be able to properly place the bands needed to hold the arch wire to move and guide the teeth.

33. D: Nerve tissue is classified as having low sensitivity to ionizing radiation. This means that when exposed to radiation, the negative effects or changes that take place to nerve tissue are minimal. It does not mean that it is safe to expose nerve tissue to radiation, because no radiation exposure is safe, but less damage can be done. Bone marrow is a type of tissue that is highly sensitive to radiation exposure and has a higher chance of being negatively impacted if exposed. Connective tissue and oral mucosa are grouped and identified to have medium sensitivity to ionizing radiation.

34. A: When the orthodontic assistant is performing procedures under direct supervision, this means that the procedures that have been authorized by the orthodontist can be done as long as the orthodontist is present in the office. The orthodontist does not need to be next to the orthodontic assistant and does not need to watch every step of the procedure, but he or she must be present in the office while it is being performed. The orthodontist must authorize every procedure that takes place in his or her practice because it is his or her license that any auxiliary staff members are working under. For procedures that fall under the direct supervision category, the orthodontist is also required to meet with and examine the patient before the patient leaves the clinic in order to review the work completed by the auxiliary staff member.

35. B: The assistant is positioned at 2 to 4 o'clock. Both the operator and the assistant must be positioned so they have a clear view of the patient's mouth. There are 4 working zones about the patient with the patient's head considered the 12 o'clock position: the operator's zone (9 to 12 o'clock), the static zone (12 to 2 o'clock), the assistant's zone (2 to 4 o'clock) and the transfer zone (4 to 9 o'clock).

36. B: Foods that are classified as cariogenic should be minimized or avoided when possible, which should be discussed with the patient. Each patient will have a different bacterial environment in his or her mouth along with a different salivary flow rate, but the one thing that does remain the same is that when cariogenic foods are introduced into the mouth, rates of dental decay increase. These include simple sugar foods such as cookies, crackers, soda, and candy.

37. C: Each type of tooth has its own specific purpose in the oral cavity. The main function of the premolars is to hold food in place as the individual is eating and then, as the food is being held by the cusp of the tooth, the other cusp of the premolar tooth grinds up the food to allow for easier digestion and processing. When these teeth are removed, their functions fall to the other teeth in the mouth, commonly the molars as they shift up to take the space that remains following the extraction of the premolars.

38. D: This is an example of abandonment—described as when an orthodontist and his or her team starts treatment on a patient but decides to stop the treatment before it is finished without request by the patient. There are many reasons why this could occur, but if a dental team decides to stop treatment, they are required by law to provide the patient with advance written notice that they are being removed as a patient from the orthodontic practice. The orthodontist must continue to see that patient even after that notice until the patient is able to find a new orthodontic practitioner.

39. B: Prehypertension is defined as a systolic blood pressure of 120–129 mmHg and/or a diastolic blood pressure of 80–89 mmHg. The dental team has the responsibility of informing the patient of these blood pressure readings and to encourage the patient to seek out his or her medical provider for further evaluation because an elevated blood pressure reading can be one of the signs of an increased risk of cardiovascular disease.

40. C: When the orthodontist is placing the bands on the back teeth, both upper and lower, pressure should be placed on the mesial and distal surfaces of the band. When this is done, the band will slide into the space created by the separators with no accidental bending or change in shape of the metal band. Each band is carefully selected and fitted to each tooth, so if there is any change in the shape of the band during placement, it can negatively affect the next steps in the process including the placement of the arch wire and movement of the teeth.

41. C: Utility wax, also called bending wax, is used to coat brackets to decrease discomfort while patients are becoming adjusted to the orthodontic appliances. Boxing wax is used to provide a barrier to keep gypsum in place before it sets. Sticky wax is used to hold broken pieces together temporarily while awaiting repair. Utility was, boxing wax, and sticky wax are all types of processing waxes. Undercut wax is used to fill undercuts before obtaining impressions.

42. C: When the orthodontic assistant is informing the orthodontist of the patient's status, it should be indicated that there is excess cement on the facial aspect of the front teeth, which is the outside area of the teeth, or the area that is found next to the lips. The lingual area of the teeth is the inside part, or the area that is found next to the tongue. The mesial and distal areas are found between the teeth.

43. C: The tray should be inserted sideways into the mouth, rotated into position, and then pressed against the teeth and seated by applying pressure from back toward the front. The orthodontic assistant must use care to avoid touching the teeth before the tray is in the correct position in the mouth. After seating, the assistant should run a finger around the mouth vestibule to make sure the lips are free and no tissue is trapped. The assistant must continue to monitor the patient for evidence of gagging, dyspnea, or choking.

44. C: In dentistry, the type of energy produced must be moving extremely fast in order to penetrate the tissues of the patient's head and neck. In order to accomplish this, the dental tubehead creates short wavelengths, meaning that there are many waves in each x-ray beam that is generated. These wavelengths must also be moving very fast, which is referred to as frequency. If the waves that are produced lack either a short wavelength or a high frequency, they will not be able to pass through the skin, jawbone, upper jaw, and other structures of the head and neck and will therefore not produce the quality of radiographs required to guide dental care.

45. C: The standard of care is the level and quality of care that patients can expect when they visit an orthodontist. This is measured by comparing other orthodontists that provide that same care in that same geographical area. If a patient seeks care in a busy urban area, the standard of care would be assessed by what other orthodontists provide in a similarly busy urban area; alternately, if a patient lives in a more rural area, the standard of care would be defined by what is common in a similar rural area. Although the standards of care may vary, they do not allow for orthodontists to practice outside of their scope or to violate basic ethical principles.

46. B: Sequential plastic aligners, which are usually changed every two to three weeks, should be worn around the clock but are removed for routine dental care, such as brushing and flossing, and while eating to prevent food for getting under the appliance. Aligners are crafted individually for patients with a computer imaging system so that they fit precisely and slowly move teeth into the correct position. The overall length of time needed for use of sequential plastic aligners and number of aligners vary depending on patients' needs.

47. D: A bite stick is the appropriate instrument that the orthodontic assistant should have prepared for the orthodontist during an appointment to place molar bands on the teeth. Once the orthodontist manually places a band around each tooth, this tool will then be used to have the patient bite down upon. This will result in the band moving into the correct position where it will remain to support the arch wire that will be used in combination with the brackets.

48. B: 7–9 years. Permanent teeth appear at various times between 6 years and 21 years, although there is a wide range and some people may experience delayed obstruction, usually because of impaction, especially of the third molars.

- Upper incisors: 7–9 years
- Lower incisors: 6–8 years
- Upper canines: 11–12 years
- Lower canines: 9–10 years
- Premolars: 10–12 years
- First molars: 6–7 years
- Second molars: 11–13 years
- Third molars: 17–21 years

49. B: The orthodontic assistant must use a fulcrum action when placing orthodontic separators. A fulcrum action is a skill that can be developed and involves the use of placing a finger or two on certain teeth to provide a resting spot for the hand, using that placement as leverage to complete fine movements in the mouth. For example, if the orthodontic assistant is placing separators between teeth #28 and #29, the pointer and middle fingers can be rested on the lower anterior teeth while placing the separators. This helps protect the assistant as well as the patient by increasing hand stability when working with sharp instruments that can easily penetrate the soft tissues of the patient's mouth. Procedures and actions including limited rinses, placing cement onto dental brackets, and exposing dental radiographs involve larger movements that take place mostly outside of the oral cavity with no opportunity to fulcrum.

50. C: Howe pliers are used to place and remove archwires. Weingart pliers may also be used for the same purpose. Prong pliers are used to adjust retainers or other active dental appliances. Edgewise pliers are used to make 90° bends. Bird Beak instruments are also used to bend wires. There are many specialized instruments and pliers used for orthodontia, including band removing and bracket removing pliers, as well as various cutters, such as distal end cutters and ligature cutters.

51. A: The dental assistant should take bitewing images, which will allow the dentist to effectively visualize between the teeth to identify any areas of decay that may be present. These include areas that are in early phases of decay so the dentist can work with the patient to implement additional preventive measure including increased flossing and fluoride treatments before the bands and brackets are placed. Periapical images are best used to view the entire tooth and ensure that the overall health of the tooth is intact, while occlusal images are used to view an entire arch on a single image.

52. C: The orthodontist assistant should set up another appointment for the patient to bring in her medications because the patient may take medications that pose increased risks, such as steroids for asthma or anticoagulants for the heart condition. Patients should be advised when they make an appointment to bring their medications or a medication list with them and should be asked detailed questions about any medications they are taking, including OTC drugs such as aspirin.

53. B: A coolant, such as air-water spray, is used with a high-speed dental handpiece because the high-speed friction against the tooth produces heat, which can result in pulpal damage. The speed, which may be up to 400,000 rpm, should be controlled with the rheostat. The bits are referred to as burs and are available in various sizes and shapes for different purposes. Most are made of tungsten carbide or diamond. High-speed dental handpieces are used to cut teeth and finish restorations.

54. C: When working with a patient, the orthodontic assistant should position themselves so that when seated their face is 12–14 inches away from the patient's. This is to reduce the strain on the assistant's neck and the eyes. If this space is less than 12 inches or greater than 14 inches, the orthodontic assistant will likely be straining the neck muscles to compensate for the incorrect distance. The eyes are also negatively affected if this distance is incorrect, possibly resulting in squinting or unnecessary stress being placed on the eyes.

55. B: HIPAA stands for the Health Insurance Portability and Accountability Act and was initiated and implemented in 1996. This act protects the privacy of patient information. If someone other than the patient would like access to a medical or dental record, the patient must sign a release to provide such access. If the patient is a minor child, the parents must provide such access, but once the patient reaches the age of 18, parents can no longer have access to those records without the consent release form being filled out by the patient. This important act is in place to protect any and all medical and dental records, and HIPAA infractions are punishable by fines and legal action.

56. D: The item that the dental team will use to cut any visible ends of the ligature wire is the pin and ligature cutter. The ligature wire goes around each bracket on each tooth. If the dental team leaves any extra wire in the mouth, the patient has a higher chance of sustaining damage to the gum tissue and other oral tissues because of the razor-sharp wire.

57. A: When preparing pastes for polysulfide impressions, first the syringe material is mixed and then the tray material. Each paste has two components, an accelerator and a base, with the accelerator dispensed first and then the base material. The two components of the syringe material are combined with the accelerator mixed into the base and the two components of the tray material are mixed about one minute later. The syringe material is loaded into the syringe chamber, and the tray material loaded into the tray with a spatula.

58. D: When the dental team uses wire ligature ties, they must ensure that a 4–5 mm long tail remains at each end after the wire is wrapped around the bracket. This will help when it comes time to remove the ligature ties and will give the staff who removes the ties something to grasp onto to initiate the removal. If the ties are any longer than 4–5 mm, it can lead to irritation and potential injury to the patient's lips, cheeks, or other soft tissue that may come into contact with the wire ligature tie.

59. D: The latent period is the time period that occurs starting from when an individual was exposed to radiation until the time that this patient developed cancer. This time period can be different because each body reacts to and processes radiation differently. The effects are cumulative, but the body can and does work to repair itself following any exposure, large or small. Often, it can be challenging to link exposures to illness due to the time that occurs between these two factors, but it should be carefully investigated and documented.

60. C: In the universal numbering system, the upper central incisors in the middle of the mouth are number 8 and 9 with number 1 the last upper molar on the right and 16 the last upper molar on the left. The last bottom molar on the left is number 17 and the last bottom molar on the right is 32. Deciduous dentition uses letters, with A the last molar on the right (EF the central upper incisors) and J, K is the last molar on the left and T the last molar on the right.

61. C: When the orthodontic assistant is performing any type of polishing procedure, these are known as class III movements. These movements include the use of the fingers, wrist, and elbow. Class I movements involve the use of the fingers only, while class II movements include the fingers and the wrist. These motions are important in the orthodontic office because they reduce the ergonomic burden that can occur by using additional parts of the body on an ongoing basis. Class IV movements are larger movements that involve everything in class III in addition to the arm and the shoulders. The dental team must focus on proper ergonomics and body mechanics in order to prevent poor habits that could lead to injury.

62. D: The face bow is a tool used in orthodontics when the orthodontist decides that, for correct orthodontic treatment, the upper first molars should move toward the back of the mouth. This will help create additional space in the arch and allow for teeth to properly grow into those spaces and avoid crowding. This is not a desirable option for many patients because it can be visually unappealing and can be challenging to wear, but with good compliance the orthodontist and patient can use this for a short time period and experience positive results that would otherwise be challenging to obtain.

63. A: After any orthodontic therapy is complete, the dental team and the patient must focus on retention so that the teeth that have been repositioned throughout the treatment do not move back to their original positions. Retention also allows for the oral structures to rest after substantial changes in teeth positioning and oral tissue changes. The type of retention will depend on the orthodontist and what is available for the patient and includes options such as the Hawley retainer, lingual retainer, positioner, and vacuum-formed retainers.

64. C: Functional occlusion refers to the type of movements in the mouth related to biting and chewing. These types of movements will change as a result of orthodontic treatment. The changes will be most noticeable during the first few days following an adjustment visit at the orthodontist and will continue to take place until the treatment is finalized. Functional occlusion will be carefully monitored by the orthodontist to ensure that it is not negatively affecting any other involved structures.

65. D: The orthodontic assistant should use the color red to chart restorations that need to be completed or those that need attention. This color is used because it brings attention when clinical staff view a patient's chart. In offices that use digital technology, many charting software solutions continue to use red to indicate teeth in electronic charts that need attention. Blue, black, and green are commonly used to indicate restorations that are present or that currently exist in the mouth, which do not need attention by the orthodontic team or the general dentistry team.

66. A: During flossing, the floss must be held taut so that the patient flossing can control the direction and pressure of flossing, so the working area (the area doing the actual flossing) should be kept at about one to one and one-half inches in length. The patient should begin with a piece of floss 18 inches long, winding one end about the left index finger and the other end about the right. As the patient flosses, he or she unwinds from one finger and winds with the other, advancing the floss.

67. A: Periapical radiographs are used to diagnose abscesses and other abnormalities, such as cysts, in the periapical region, especially with a film holder and the paralleling technique. Multiple views may be required to adequately diagnose an abnormality. Bitewing radiographs are useful for proximal caries, showing molars but not the apical regions. Occlusal films are used to evaluate the submandibular glands and impacted canine teeth (upper). Posteroanterior radiographs are used to diagnose trauma in the skull or facial bones.

68. D: The extra area of enamel found on the inside of these upper first molars is referred to as the cusp of Carabelli. This is a normal anatomical feature of the two upper first molars and should be taken into consideration when bands need to be placed on these teeth to ensure that the bands have the proper fit. This feature will not be present on the lower teeth and does not need to be accounted for when selecting those bands. The cingulum, lingual ridge, and fossa are other normal anatomical structures and features that are common on anterior teeth, both primary and permanent, but they have less consideration in orthodontics because they are found on the lingual surface of the front teeth, with minimal need to manipulate those areas.

69. C: The radial artery is found on the inner surface of the wrist on the side of the thumb. It is commonly used to record the patient's heart rate during a dental examination. If the dental team cannot find a pulse in this location, they can also try the carotid artery found on the outside of the neck or the brachial artery found on the inner surface of the forearm. The heart rate is one of the common measurements that is monitored, in addition to the patient's respiratory rate and blood pressure at the start of each appointment.

70. C: Penumbra is the name of the blurriness that the orthodontist is indicating as being present on each of the bitewing images. This can occur when the exposure factors are not correct and can result in the images needing to be recaptured if the penumbra is affecting the orthodontist's ability to provide a proper diagnosis. In order to prevent dental images from becoming blurry, the dental team must have their machines calibrated according to the manufacturer's directions, must prevent patient movement during imaging, and must use digital sensors that are known for their ability to provide clear images. An image with penumbra will not always need to be recaptured; the dental team can make this decision.

71. A: When cementing and placing bands onto the teeth, the dental team needs to ensure that the teeth are dried off and protected against moisture. If the teeth become contaminated during the placement procedure, it could compromise the strength of the band cement. The band should be held on the top and the bottom versus the sides of the surface to prevent distortion with the side that will be placed next to the gum tissue facing upward for proper placement by the orthodontist. Once the orthodontist places the band, the assistant will transfer an instrument called the band seater to the orthodontist and the dental team will have the patient close down and bite gently onto the band, allowing for gentle guidance into the correct area on the tooth.

72. D: Headgear tubes are cylindrical-type tubes that are round in shape and are placed on the bands that go on the first molars. These tubes are used by the orthodontist when it is known that the patient may need to wear headgear; they help the orthodontist to use the face-bow appliance during the fitting of the headgear.

73. D: Veracity is one of the basic ethical principles that must be followed in dentistry; it involves being honest and telling the truth to all patients. Often, a patient may select a different option than what the orthodontist prefers for various reasons, including cost. If the patient is only provided with the option(s) that the orthodontist prefers, that is a violation of veracity, which is an important component in building and maintaining the patient and dental team relationship.

74. D: Dental sealants are a very important part of dentistry that help prevent decay from starting on the teeth. A sealant can be placed on the permanent teeth as soon as they erupt in the mouth. It is applied in a thick liquid form so that it enters into any deep crevices that are found on the biting surfaces of the teeth, and then it hardens—essentially blocking out any room for bacteria, food, or other particles to enter into these areas and cause decay. The orthodontic team should be knowledgeable of this preventive option so that sealants can be recommended to their patients as new teeth erupt in the dentition.

75. A: When a patient is exposed to a panoramic image, the tubehead part of the panoramic machine will rotate behind the patient and the digital plates will rotate in front of the patient's head. This differs from standard dental imaging in which the tubehead is placed on the side or in front of the patient and remains there during the exposure. The beam that results from panoramic imaging is very small and resembles a vertical slit versus a circular beam of 2.75 inches that is produced when using a circular position indicating device for periapical and bitewing images. The panoramic machine imaging process lasts for up to 10 seconds and must not be stopped during exposure because distortion to the image will occur.

76. D: When orthodontists smooth out the structure that the brackets have been bonded to for an orthodontic procedure, they may often use a high- or slow-speed handpiece and remove a very thin layer of the enamel along with the residual bonding material. If the orthodontist removes too much of the enamel, there is a risk of exposure of the dentin, which lies directly under the enamel. This can cause increased sensitivity due to the nerves in the dentin being exposed, while also being visually unappealing for the patient because the dentin is yellow in color versus the white enamel. The coronal pulp is found in the upper part of the tooth, with the apical foramen and radicular fibers being found in the roots of the teeth.

77. B: Teeth that have been circled in red are teeth that are present yet not visible in the mouth due to a lack of eruption. It is important to know that they are still present in the mouth because they could grow in and affect the orthodontic treatment. The timing of the expected eruption of these teeth may affect the placement of any orthodontics. These teeth are commonly identified by reviewing radiographic images. Teeth that have been extracted should be crossed out with a black or blue "x" to indicate that the tooth is no longer part of the patient's dentition. If a tooth needs to be removed, it should be crossed out with a red "x" to indicate that action is needed. It is important to note if crowns are present in the mouth as well so they can be factored in to the orthodontic treatment. The charting notations for crowns vary according to the materials that they are made from.

78. A: Radiographic screening should follow history and physical exam and should never precede the exam to ensure that the correct screening is conducted and to avoid unnecessary exposure to radiation. Additionally, the status of returning patients may have changed. All radiographs should be carefully examined for evidence of caries, periodontal disease, or other disorders. Intraoral radiographs should be used for evaluation of the teeth and alveoli while extraoral radiographs should be used for concerns outside of this complex.

79. C: The orthodontic assistant is performing a procedure that is outside of the legal scope of practice for the assistant, resulting in a violation of criminal law. State dental boards provide various informational materials that describe the scope of practice for each type of dental provider or auxiliary staff member, and it is law that all staff are aware of and abide by these materials. The orthodontic team cannot justify going outside of their scope because of being short staffed or not knowing what was illegal to perform. In this case, the orthodontist and the orthodontic assistant could have charges brought against them and may have any applicable dental licenses suspended or revoked.

80. C: The orthodontist will place the bands on the upper and lower first and second molars. These teeth provide the most structure and support for these bands and will serve as the base for the orthodontic treatment. Often, the premolars and anterior teeth need to be moved throughout the treatment; therefore, placing bands in these locations would prevent the teeth from receiving the pressure from the bands correctly. The bands will then serve as the location that holds the arch wire into place to guide the movement of the teeth.

81. D: Separating pliers are used to stretch the elastic separators so they can be placed between the teeth. The separator is placed over the points of the pliers, then the pliers squeezed to open and stretch the elastic, which is seated between the teeth in a back and forth maneuver, similar to that used when flossing. Once the separator is in place, the pliers are removed. Alternately, a separator can be placed by looping two strands of dental floss through the separator, grasping the ends of the floss on both sides, and then pulling in opposite directions to stretch out the separator.

82. A: These symptoms are consistent with acute hypoglycemia, which can result from excess insulin or inadequate food intake, causing the blood glucose level to fall below 50–60 mg/dL. Patients may exhibit a range of symptoms, including seizures, altered consciousness, lethargy, myoclonus, respiratory distress, diaphoresis, hypothermia, aggression, agitation, cyanosis, diaphoresis, tremor, tachycardia, palpitation, hunger, and anxiety. Immediate treatment includes providing glucose, such as 4 lumps of sugar or a drink high in glucose.

83. C: The name given to this type of bite is called crossbite. This can be described as a type of malposition that results when teeth that should be more toward the outer surface (toward the cheek) are instead found closer to the tongue. In this patient's case, the upper premolars are located more lingual than they should be and the lower premolars are located more buccal than they should be. This can result in a displeasing aesthetic because it can be seen when the patient smiles. This condition can be corrected through various types of orthodontic therapy.

84. A: 110 pliers are also referred to as Howe pliers. These are used in almost all orthodontic procedures that use brackets and bands, and they help prepare the arch wire for being placed into the bands where it will start the process of moving the teeth into the desired positions.

85. C: Patients should be apprised of all reasonable risks and any complications or adverse effects, such as post-procedure pain, as well as benefits. Providing informed consent is a requirement of all states. Informed consent must be signed by the patient or guardian prior to procedures and should include:

- Explanation of diagnosis
- Nature of, and reason for, treatment or procedure
- Risks and benefits
- Alternative options (regardless of cost or insurance coverage)
- Risks and benefits of alternative options
- Risks and benefits of not having a treatment or procedure

86. C: The adult teeth that will eventually replace the baby teeth or the primary teeth are classified as succedaneous. These teeth will succeed, or replace, the baby teeth that fall out as the permanent teeth grow in, push on, and displace the roots of the baby teeth. Mixed dentition is when the patient has baby teeth and adult teeth present, while deciduous and primary dentition are other names for baby teeth.

87. A: When placing elastomeric separators, the orthodontic assistant must use a back-and-forth, or seesaw, motion with the separator to gently maneuver it between the teeth. This allows for a small amount of the separator to slide through the contacts; over time, the entire separator will fall into place in the embrasure space. The orthodontic assistant should not use pressure or roughly pull the separator into the proximal space nor have the patient bite into the separator, which could damage the patient's oral tissue. Pointed instruments such as the explorer should not be used for placement because their use increases the risk of puncturing the oral tissue.

88. D: The dental team is noticing an error that is created when the vertical angle of the dental tubehead is incorrect. When there is too large of a vertical angle, this causes the biting area of the teeth to not appear on the radiograph, whereas too small of an angle causes the root tips to be absent on the dental radiograph. These are common errors that occur when capturing periapical images and can be corrected by additional training. When the side-to-side movement of the tubehead is incorrect, it can lead to blurred areas between the teeth; when the tubehead is not placed over the sensor, it can lead to a white circular area appearing on the images.

89. B: The orthodontic assistant should immediately begin CPR with 30 chest compressions at 100/min followed by 2 ventilations (30:2) and should not delay while the AED is obtained. The compressions-only protocol is intended for untrained/nonmedical bystanders, and all compressions are now done at the rate of 100/min. After initial cycles, the assistant can procure the AED if one is nearby and follow procedures for shocking, repeating every 2 minutes with resumption of CPR in between shocks. If a bag mask is available, then ventilation can be done about every 10 compressions.

90. A: Oral candidiasis (thrush) is a fungal infection that can occur in the mouth, especially in those who are immunocompromised (such as AIDS patients and those receiving chemotherapy). Symptoms include white cheesy-appearing lesions, which may bleed if they are disturbed and may cover the entire oral cavity including the tongue, inside of cheeks, palate, and gums. Candidiasis is painful and often associated with loss of taste. Candidiasis may be treated with antifungal medications. Non-sweetened yogurt and acidophilus may be consumed to help prevent candidiasis.

91. B: The correct chart notation to use for impacted teeth is to encircle the entire tooth in red. This is a universal notation that informs the treating dentist that these teeth are present but they have not yet become visible nor have they erupted into the oral cavity. This is important for orthodontists to know because if these teeth grow in unexpectedly during orthodontic treatment, it may shift the treatment plan as they take up a substantial amount of room in the oral cavity and therefore must be accounted for during the initial exam.

92. D: The orthodontic team should recommend toothpaste with hydrogen peroxide as the active ingredient for patients who are asking about a whitening toothpaste. Hydrogen peroxide along with carbamide peroxide are the active ingredients that are responsible for breaking down tough stains and providing whitening results for patients when used as the manufacturer recommends. Often, these toothpastes are used in combination with other whitening products as a way to achieve desired whitening results for patients who have finished orthodontic treatment.

93. D: In recent years, a new type of three-dimensional imaging has become available in dentistry called cone beam computed tomography, which allows the dental team to see the structures on a given image in three dimensions. This allows for a deeper understanding of the structures present on the film and their anatomical placement and provides an image with much more detail compared to the standard two-dimensional forms of dental imaging including the common intraoral periapical image, bitewing image, and extraoral panoramic image.

94. B: The thyroid gland is one of the four organs of the body that are identified as critical organs. The skin, lens of the eye, and the bone marrow in the head and neck region are the remaining three critical organs. When exposed to radiation, these areas have the potential to be affected; if that occurs, the results can be very damaging to the patient. These are also areas that are frequently exposed to radiation in dentistry due to the nature of the head and neck regions that are examined. Safety precautions have been developed and should always be followed when exposing critical organs including the use of the thyroid collar, the paralleling technique, and the correct prescription protocol for dental images.

95. B: Tooth #30 is found in the lower right quadrant according to the universal numbering system, which is commonly used in general dentistry and in orthodontics. Other teeth found in this quadrant include teeth #25–32. Although not all of the teeth in that range are always present, anytime the orthodontist indicates one of those numbers, the assistant should know they will be found in the lower right quadrant.

96. A: The orthodontic scaler is an instrument that would be appropriate to include in the tray setup for the removal of elastomeric rings from an orthodontic patient. This instrument has a small working end that resembles a hook that can easily be inserted into the edge of an elastomeric band and then gently pulls out the band with pressure. While the orthodontic assistant is removing the band, the fingers can be placed over the scaler and the band to prevent trauma to the tissue if it comes out quicker than expected.

97. A: By not renewing the national certification that is required in their state of employment, orthodontic assistants can be cited for an infraction, which could result in fees being incurred and could even result in a suspension of an assistant's certification depending on the certifying agency. The orthodontic assistant's certification status could be detected in an annual certification audit or may be noted when the assistant attempts to renew the expired certification. For this reason, renewal notices are sent out far in advance so that dental team members can renew their respective credentials in a timely manner.

98. A: The bracket holds the arch wire in place on each tooth. It is cemented onto each tooth and has small grooves where the arch wire will fit in when it is placed. The dental team will then use a metal or plastic tie to hold the arch wire in place on each tooth. Resin can be used to cement the brackets into place if desired by the dental team, but it is often not the first choice.

99. B: The temporalis raises the jaw and is associated with temporomandibular joint (TMJ) syndrome. Misalignment, grinding or clenching the teeth can stress the joint and put pressure on the nerves that pass through the neck and jaw, resulting in pain. The masseter raises the jaw and controls the rate at which the jaw falls open. The medial pterygoid closes the jaw and moves it laterally. The lateral pterygoid opens the mouth, allows protrusion and lateral movement of the mandible.

100. C: The correct sequence is separator placement, band placement, bonding of brackets, arch wire, and then adjustment checks. The separators are used first because these will create space between the teeth for the bands to be placed. Otherwise, the bands would not fit in the spaces between the teeth. Once the bands are placed, the dental team can then select and bond on or cement on the brackets. These are the areas into which the arch wire will be inserted, so the brackets must be cemented on prior to the arch wire being placed. Finally, the patient will come in on a recurring basis for adjustment checks.

101. A: One of the main functions of saliva is to help clear food particles within the oral cavity during and after chewing. The saliva that automatically enters the mouth during the sight, smell, or introduction of food into the mouth provides important support in mixing with the food particles that are being consumed and in helping to swallow the food. Saliva in the mouth also helps remove any food buildup or plaque that can remain on the teeth after eating. If a patient indicates not having adequate saliva, the orthodontic team can discuss various dental aids that can help to increase the rate of saliva production.

102. B: The Hawley retainer is a very common type of retainer that is created following the completion of orthodontic therapy. Its role is to hold the teeth in position and prevent any movement once the braces or other type of treatments are removed. This type of retainer can be taken in and out of the mouth and is made of a resin type of material. It should be worn as much as possible while the tooth structures and gingival tissue heal and rebuild in their new positions following treatment.

103. B: The orthodontic team must review the dental and medical records of each patient prior to the patient's appointment—this step helps prevent unexpected medical emergencies from occurring and familiarizes the orthodontist and the dental team with the specific patient and his or her individual needs. Sterilized (not simply disinfected) dental instruments should be available for use and should be set out within the pouches they were sterilized in along with the supplies that will be used for the procedure prior to the patient entering the treatment room. By having the items that will be used out and ready, and leaving them in their packaging, the dental team can save valuable setup time and the patient can see that the items are in sterile packaging and watch the dental team open them. It is important for the billing team to collect insurance and payment information prior to the visit so the patient is aware of his or her portion of any costs resulting from the visit. This information can take time for the dental team to obtain from the insurance company and is a valuable step in ensuring financial transparency with the patient.

104. B: The best method for examining the dorsal (upper) surface of the tongue is to ask the patient to protrude the tongue. The tongue can then be grasped with gauze so that it can be held for examination, as the posterior one-third is difficult to visualize otherwise. When examining the floor of the mouth and the ventral surface, the orthodontic assistant should ask the patient to push the tongue toward a cheek, first one side and then the other.

105. C: The equivalent to the roentgen in the International System of Units measuring system is the coulomb per kilogram. Both of these units measure the amount of radiation that a given patient is exposed to in a specific environment. The traditional system of measurement is still commonly used but was more prevalent in the past. The International System of Units, or Système Internationale, is the newer system that many scientists who study radiation exposure use to report their data. To ensure that the dental team can use both systems, equivalents have been identified; therefore, regardless of the system used, the dental team can interpret results to any radiation testing that may occur in their dental office.

106. C: Occlusal radiographs provide a view of the palate and the mouth floor and are indicated to identify supernumerary teeth because this type of imaging shows skeletal anatomy. The film is placed between the upper and lower teeth (on the occlusal surfaces) and the patient bites gently to hold the film in place. The film may be placed front to back or side to side, depending on the area of concern. A mandibular projection is used to visualize the floor of the mouth and impacted lower teeth or fractures and a maxillary projection for the palate and maxillary sinus.

107. A: When the orthodontic assistant and the orthodontist are properly seated, the transfer of instruments should take place in the 7–12 o'clock zone. This is the location that will produce the least amount of ergonomic strain on the orthodontist and the orthodontic assistant by minimizing arm and elbow movements that are involved in instrument transfer; it will also prevent them from having to reach for an instrument during the transfer. The orthodontic assistant must work to set up the treatment room so that this positioning and transfer zone can be accomplished as directed by the orthodontist.

108. A: While individual preferences in setting up trays may vary somewhat, generally armamentarium should be placed according to sequence of use, starting from the left and going to the right, and instruments are usually also grouped according to function. Hinged instruments (such as hemostats) may be placed on the right. Cotton supplies (wadding, rolls, etc.) are usually placed across the tray top for easy access. Once an instrument is used and returned to the assistant, it should be replaced in its initial position.

109. B: Gemination: a tooth abnormality in which one developing tooth partially divides into two teeth. Fusion: an abnormality in which two adjacent developing teeth fuse together into one tooth. Dens invaginatus: an abnormality in which the outside of the tooth folds inward, creating a fold that appears as though the tooth contains a smaller tooth inside of it. Concrescence: an abnormality in which two adjacent developing teeth fuse together in their cementum, usually because of overcrowding.

110. D: The lingual retainer is made of light steel wire. It is a permanent retainer that cannot be removed once placed because it is cemented on with a very strong material. This retainer is placed from the lower left canine to the lower right canine and is commonly used on the lower arch immediately following the removal of the brackets and any other orthodontic treatment. This is a type of retention that will allow for the bone to remold itself following treatment as well as the gum tissue to heal and build to surround the tooth structures in their new positions.

111. C: The orthodontic assistant is having the patient bite into the notched area to ensure that the patient's focal trough imaging layer is correctly aligned. Correct alignment ensures that the patient's anatomy is positioned appropriately, allowing for the machine to capture an image that can be read and diagnosed by the orthodontist. If the patient is biting outside of this notched area, the focal trough will be off, representing an incorrect anatomical position during the exposure, resulting in distorted and blurred images.

112. A: Xylitol is a sugar substitute that has been found to decrease the risk of tooth decay, which makes it a good choice for the orthodontic team to recommend to patients who are undergoing orthodontic therapy. The recommendation can be for patients to consume sweets and other products that contain xylitol versus the same types of products that contain sugar in its natural form or other sugar substitutes. Of note, the use of xylitol does not remove the need for brushing and flossing of the teeth as recommended by the orthodontic and general dentistry teams.

113. C: Before the dental team can cement on the brackets used for traditional braces, they must clean the teeth with pumice using a prophy cup. This motion of the cup and the abrasiveness of the pumice will prepare the enamel tissue to properly bond to the cement and the bracket. If this cleaning does not take place, the brackets will still adhere to the teeth but could come off prematurely, causing inconvenience for the patient and delays in orthodontic progress.

114. B: Vacuum-formed clear aligners are a very popular new option in orthodontics, providing a way for the teeth to be moved into their desired positions without the need for the metal braces that have traditionally been used in orthodontics. Unlike traditional braces, the aligners can be removed during treatment in situations such as brushing and eating but must be placed immediately back on to obtain the desired tooth movement. This can be challenging for some patients who may want to remove the aligners on a more frequent basis, resulting in delayed movement and longer treatment. The dental patient visits the dental office frequently to obtain new aligners to continue to move the teeth until the end of the treatment is reached.

115. C: This notation refers to the lower left central incisor. Decidious teeth are lettered from the central incisors, both upper and lower, starting with letter A, B, C, D, and ending with the last molar at E.

- ⌈A This symbol in front of a letter indicates lower left.
- A⌉ This symbol behind a letter indicates lower right.
- ⌊A This symbol in front of a letter indicates upper left.
- A⌋ This symbol behind the letter indicates upper right.

116. B: Chronic radiation exposure occurs when a dental team member is exposed to small amounts of radiation over a prolonged period of time. This could happen due to not following the required safety precautions including standing too close to the tubehead during exposure or not standing behind a wall with the appropriate shielding barriers to prevent radiation exposure. These small amounts daily or weekly over years can lead to biological changes in the exposed individual years or decades later, and it is difficult to correlate them to a specific exposure setting or event.

117. B: The dental team can inform the caregiver and the patient that these molars typically erupt on the top arch at approximately ages 12–13, although this timeline may vary. On the bottom, they may erupt as early as age 11. The final teeth to come in following these second molars will be the third molars, which will not typically start to present until age 17.

118. B: During the check-in portion of the examination, the blood pressure, pulse (heart rate), and respiratory rate are commonly measured. If a patient presents to an appointment directly after engaging in physical activity, the dental team can expect an increased pulse, respiratory rate, and blood pressure. This is the body's natural response to get more oxygen to the tissues in the body to support increased cardiovascular effort. The dental team should note any increases and also note the physical exercise that the patient was engaged in prior to the examination.

119. C: When the orthodontic assistant is preparing to provide patient care, his or her thighs should be positioned parallel to the floor with the knees being lower than the hips. This positioning will reduce any strain on the thighs and the knees and will help blood flow in the lower extremities to remain uninterrupted while sitting. The orthodontic assistant should always place his or her feet flat on the floor, have the backrest supporting the lower back, and be seated as far back on the dental chair as possible.

120. A: By not participating in the negative conversations about or toward other staff and patients, the orthodontic assistant is demonstrating the basic ethical principle of nonmaleficence (aka doing no harm). When staff talk negatively about other staff members, it can create a stressful and toxic work environment. This can cause harm to the relationships that are formed with staff who work together on a daily basis and may ultimately impact patient care.

121. A: The Council on Radiation Protection and Measurements has set the limits for dental team members at 5 rem per year for occupational exposure to ionizing radiation. This is based on the study of how radiation affects the body and the doses that are needed to cause biological changes. The dental team has the ability to measure radiation exposure by wearing a radiation monitoring badge that can be sent out to an external company for interpretation, with the results then being reported back to the dental office. Annual results that total <5 rem per year are acceptable. Anything over this limit would require mitigation for the overexposure.

122. A: When the orthodontic assistant is transferring a hinged-type instrument, including posterior band removal pliers, it should always be transferred with the handle portion being placed into the orthodontist's palm. The pliers should be in the closed position, and a two-handed technique can be used if needed due to the weight of some hinged orthodontic instruments. Proper instrument transfers allow for a smooth procedure and a positive patient experience, often minimizing the amount of time needed for the appointment.

123. B: The orthodontic assistant should recommend that non-milk extrinsic sugars, which include glucose and sucrose, be consumed only during mealtimes with other foods and restricted to no more than 4 servings per day. Intrinsic sugars are found in fruits and vegetables and are much healthier for the teeth and extrinsic sugars, so children should be provided 5–6 servings per day of foods containing intrinsic sugars. These foods are high in fiber and less likely to result in caries.

124. A: This type of bite is called an overbite, which can be described as the top front teeth covering most or all of the bottom front teeth when the patient bites them together. This can cause damage to the teeth and the gum tissue and can be corrected by orthodontic intervention. This differs from overjet, in which the top front teeth stick out toward the lips, a condition that can also be corrected by orthodontics.

125. C: When considering the use of ligature ties, the orthodontic assistant must know that when placing these ties, the procedure must start in the back of the mouth and then move toward the front. This will ensure that each ligature tie is in the correct positioning and will help take care of the more difficult placements in the beginning of this procedure. These ties are made of stainless steel and are a 0.01-inch thickness. Anything thicker than that would make these ties difficult to place. They can be applied on each tooth as an individual tie, or they can be tied to multiple teeth at a time, creating a chain effect. Ligature ties are commonly placed by the orthodontic assistant using ligature tying pliers.

126. D: The system that the dentist is using is known as the universal numbering system, in which each tooth is given a number, even teeth that are not yet erupted. The numbers range from 1 to 32, and the numbering starts in the upper right area of the mouth, moves to the upper left, drops down to the lower left, and then moves over to the lower right. This is a very simple and common numbering system and is used throughout dental practices both domestically and internationally, serving as a basis for understanding the locations of each tooth.

127. B: The dental tubehead is composed of many different parts that all work together and result in the production of radiation. Inside the tubehead, there is oil that takes the heat that is created when the exposure button is pressed and disseminates it throughout the oil, which resultingly maintains the dental tubehead at room temperature. Without this insulating oil, the large amounts of energy produced during image production would cause the tubehead to become hot to the touch. The metal housing maintains the integrity of the tubehead allowing for the transformers to serve their purpose and drive the radiation production inside of the dental x-ray tube.

128. B: Patients undergoing orthodontic treatment should continue to go to his or her general dentist and receive topical fluoride treatments at preventive visits. The brackets and bonding agents that are on the teeth can bring about food and plaque accumulation, which can weaken the enamel covering of the teeth. The minerals found in topical fluoride treatments serve to strengthen the enamel layer by adding minerals that have been lost due to external factors.

129. A: When placing the arch wire, the dental team must center the wire in the patient's oral cavity. This is done by lining up the mark on the arch wire with the upper front teeth, #8 and #9, using the universal numbering system. The arch wire will then fit into the buccal tubes that are found on the bands located on the back teeth. The wire should not pass out of those tubes because it will then irritate and potentially damage the oral tissue. To prevent injury and irritation during the initial placement of the wire, the dental team should measure the wire before it is placed into the mouth, allowing for it to be adequately trimmed before placement.

130. D: The assistant's stool should be positioned 4–6 inches above the height of the orthodontist's chair and as close as possible to the patient's side, with the seat about level with the patient's mouth. The assistant must have good visibility and be able to easily reach the patient's mouth and transfer instruments. The cart or tray is placed over the assistant's upper legs so that the assistant can easily reach items.

131. C: When the orthodontic assistant is measuring a patient's blood pressure, it is essential to position the patient in the correct position to obtain an accurate reading. This position includes having the patient in an upright position, similar to the supine position. The patient's arms should be at the sides, and the legs and ankles should remain uncrossed throughout the measurement. This positioning will allow for the blood to flow readily without obstructing the reading and to allow the dental team to obtain the most accurate reading possible.

132. B: In orthodontics, the team must obtain written informed consent if they are going to start any type of procedure that takes longer than 1 year to complete. There are many short procedures that are offered in orthodontics that may include the placement of a space maintainer, dental impressions for retainers, and the images needed for proper diagnosis. Although these procedures do require informed consent, it is not required to be written. It is commonly standard practice to capture a patient's consent for all treatments, but it is not legally required like it is for procedures taking longer than 1 year to complete.

133. A: The orthodontic assistant is witnessing the presence of a supernumerary (extra) tooth. This can be caused by a number of different developmental anomalies that take place during tooth formation through gemination or fusion. A single supernumerary tooth can appear, or multiple supernumerary teeth can be present throughout the mouth. These can be identified and charted as part of the patient's radiographic examination as well as the visual examination. If the supernumerary teeth affect the desired orthodontic treatment or results, they can be extracted to allow for additional space.

134. D: Children are naturally curious and apprehensive about things they are unfamiliar with, so the best initial approach is to show the child the equipment and how it works and let the child handle the equipment as much as possible. For example, the child can raise and lower the chair a few times and suction water from a cup. These activities help the child learn what to expect during the procedure and prepare the child for the accompanying noises, which can be frightening to children.

135. C: When using no-mix chemical cure adhesive for bonding of a bracket to a tooth, primer is placed on both but the paste is then placed only on the base of the bracket. While this is easier to use than two-part chemical cures, which require mixing, the no-mix adhesive has lower bond strength and a very short working time (usually about 30 to 45 seconds). It cures within 5 minutes without a curing light.

136. D: When the orthodontic assistant places elastomeric separators, they are left in place for up to 2 weeks. This allows the teeth to adequately separate and provide the space needed for the bands that will be placed on the back teeth for the next step in the orthodontic treatment. If the separators are taken out too early, the teeth can shift back into their normal positions making it difficult to place the orthodontic bands.

137. A: The described effects are known as somatic effects. These negative side effects of radiation may occur in the individual receiving radiation, but they will not be passed on to future generations. Somatic tissues include all nonreproductive tissues in the body. These tissues do experience negative effects at varying levels following radiation exposure; however, they are not passed on to future offspring.

138. A: The type of material that the orthodontic assistant is seeking to use is elastic chain ties. This is a product that is very common in orthodontics and is made of an elastic or stretchable type of plastic material making this a very easy item to place. Elastic chain ties can go onto brackets individually or can be put on in a chain-type formation where they are applied to each bracket but are connected, making them very efficient to place and preventing the need for the orthodontic assistant to have multiple pieces of elastic material available for use. This material comes in multiple colors and is commonly placed with a ligature director tool or an orthodontic scaler.

139. A: The triangular space that is formed when two teeth touch each other is called the embrasure. This space is covered by gum tissue and must be flossed to remove any particles that may be present as a result of eating food. This space is hidden by gum tissue unless the gum tissue is in the process of receding; it is then that this space will become visible. Flossing into this space is an important part of the preventive care that must be reviewed with orthodontic patients to prevent interproximal decay.

140. A: There is no safe amount of radiation exposure. All radiation has the potential to cause damage to human tissues. Because of this, there are safety requirements that must be adhered to in the dental office. One safety requirement is that the orthodontic assistant must have distance between themselves and the dental tubehead where the radiation is produced. If the orthodontic assistant stands at a minimum of 6 feet from the tubehead, any extra radiation will dissipate before it reaches the dental team member.

How to Overcome Test Anxiety

Just the thought of taking a test is enough to make most people a little nervous. A test is an important event that can have a long-term impact on your future, so it's important to take it seriously and it's natural to feel anxious about performing well. But just because anxiety is normal, that doesn't mean that it's helpful in test taking, or that you should simply accept it as part of your life. Anxiety can have a variety of effects. These effects can be mild, like making you feel slightly nervous, or severe, like blocking your ability to focus or remember even a simple detail.

If you experience test anxiety—whether severe or mild—it's important to know how to beat it. To discover this, first you need to understand what causes test anxiety.

Causes of Test Anxiety

While we often think of anxiety as an uncontrollable emotional state, it can actually be caused by simple, practical things. One of the most common causes of test anxiety is that a person does not feel adequately prepared for their test. This feeling can be the result of many different issues such as poor study habits or lack of organization, but the most common culprit is time management. Starting to study too late, failing to organize your study time to cover all of the material, or being distracted while you study will mean that you're not well prepared for the test. This may lead to cramming the night before, which will cause you to be physically and mentally exhausted for the test. Poor time management also contributes to feelings of stress, fear, and hopelessness as you realize you are not well prepared but don't know what to do about it.

Other times, test anxiety is not related to your preparation for the test but comes from unresolved fear. This may be a past failure on a test, or poor performance on tests in general. It may come from comparing yourself to others who seem to be performing better or from the stress of living up to expectations. Anxiety may be driven by fears of the future—how failure on this test would affect your educational and career goals. These fears are often completely irrational, but they can still negatively impact your test performance.

Elements of Test Anxiety

As mentioned earlier, test anxiety is considered to be an emotional state, but it has physical and mental components as well. Sometimes you may not even realize that you are suffering from test anxiety until you notice the physical symptoms. These can include trembling hands, rapid heartbeat, sweating, nausea, and tense muscles. Extreme anxiety may lead to fainting or vomiting. Obviously, any of these symptoms can have a negative impact on testing. It is important to recognize them as soon as they begin to occur so that you can address the problem before it damages your performance.

The mental components of test anxiety include trouble focusing and inability to remember learned information. During a test, your mind is on high alert, which can help you recall information and stay focused for an extended period of time. However, anxiety interferes with your mind's natural processes, causing you to blank out, even on the questions you know well. The strain of testing during anxiety makes it difficult to stay focused, especially on a test that may take several hours. Extreme anxiety can take a huge mental toll, making it difficult not only to recall test information but even to understand the test questions or pull your thoughts together.

Effects of Test Anxiety

Test anxiety is like a disease—if left untreated, it will get progressively worse. Anxiety leads to poor performance, and this reinforces the feelings of fear and failure, which in turn lead to poor performances on subsequent tests. It can grow from a mild nervousness to a crippling condition. If allowed to progress, test anxiety can have a big impact on your schooling, and consequently on your future.

Test anxiety can spread to other parts of your life. Anxiety on tests can become anxiety in any stressful situation, and blanking on a test can turn into panicking in a job situation. But fortunately, you don't have to let anxiety rule your testing and determine your grades. There are a number of relatively simple steps you can take to move past anxiety and function normally on a test and in the rest of life.

Physical Steps for Beating Test Anxiety

While test anxiety is a serious problem, the good news is that it can be overcome. It doesn't have to control your ability to think and remember information. While it may take time, you can begin taking steps today to beat anxiety.

Just as your first hint that you may be struggling with anxiety comes from the physical symptoms, the first step to treating it is also physical. Rest is crucial for having a clear, strong mind. If you are tired, it is much easier to give in to anxiety. But if you establish good sleep habits, your body and mind will be ready to perform optimally, without the strain of exhaustion. Additionally, sleeping well helps you to retain information better, so you're more likely to recall the answers when you see the test questions.

Getting good sleep means more than going to bed on time. It's important to allow your brain time to relax. Take study breaks from time to time so it doesn't get overworked, and don't study right before bed. Take time to rest your mind before trying to rest your body, or you may find it difficult to fall asleep.

Along with sleep, other aspects of physical health are important in preparing for a test. Good nutrition is vital for good brain function. Sugary foods and drinks may give a burst of energy but this burst is followed by a crash, both physically and emotionally. Instead, fuel your body with protein and vitamin-rich foods.

Also, drink plenty of water. Dehydration can lead to headaches and exhaustion, especially if your brain is already under stress from the rigors of the test. Particularly if your test is a long one, drink water during the breaks. And if possible, take an energy-boosting snack to eat between sections.

Along with sleep and diet, a third important part of physical health is exercise. Maintaining a steady workout schedule is helpful, but even taking 5-minute study breaks to walk can help get your blood pumping faster and clear your head. Exercise also releases endorphins, which contribute to a positive feeling and can help combat test anxiety.

When you nurture your physical health, you are also contributing to your mental health. If your body is healthy, your mind is much more likely to be healthy as well. So take time to rest, nourish your body with healthy food and water, and get moving as much as possible. Taking these physical steps will make you stronger and more able to take the mental steps necessary to overcome test anxiety.

Mental Steps for Beating Test Anxiety

Working on the mental side of test anxiety can be more challenging, but as with the physical side, there are clear steps you can take to overcome it. As mentioned earlier, test anxiety often stems from lack of preparation, so the obvious solution is to prepare for the test. Effective studying may be the most important weapon you have for beating test anxiety, but you can and should employ several other mental tools to combat fear.

First, boost your confidence by reminding yourself of past success—tests or projects that you aced. If you're putting as much effort into preparing for this test as you did for those, there's no reason you should expect to fail here. Work hard to prepare; then trust your preparation.

Second, surround yourself with encouraging people. It can be helpful to find a study group, but be sure that the people you're around will encourage a positive attitude. If you spend time with others who are anxious or cynical, this will only contribute to your own anxiety. Look for others who are motivated to study hard from a desire to succeed, not from a fear of failure.

Third, reward yourself. A test is physically and mentally tiring, even without anxiety, and it can be helpful to have something to look forward to. Plan an activity following the test, regardless of the outcome, such as going to a movie or getting ice cream.

When you are taking the test, if you find yourself beginning to feel anxious, remind yourself that you know the material. Visualize successfully completing the test. Then take a few deep, relaxing breaths and return to it. Work through the questions carefully but with confidence, knowing that you are capable of succeeding.

Developing a healthy mental approach to test taking will also aid in other areas of life. Test anxiety affects more than just the actual test—it can be damaging to your mental health and even contribute to depression. It's important to beat test anxiety before it becomes a problem for more than testing.

Study Strategy

Being prepared for the test is necessary to combat anxiety, but what does being prepared look like? You may study for hours on end and still not feel prepared. What you need is a strategy for test prep. The next few pages outline our recommended steps to help you plan out and conquer the challenge of preparation.

STEP 1: SCOPE OUT THE TEST

Learn everything you can about the format (multiple choice, essay, etc.) and what will be on the test. Gather any study materials, course outlines, or sample exams that may be available. Not only will this help you to prepare, but knowing what to expect can help to alleviate test anxiety.

STEP 2: MAP OUT THE MATERIAL

Look through the textbook or study guide and make note of how many chapters or sections it has. Then divide these over the time you have. For example, if a book has 15 chapters and you have five days to study, you need to cover three chapters each day. Even better, if you have the time, leave an extra day at the end for overall review after you have gone through the material in depth.

If time is limited, you may need to prioritize the material. Look through it and make note of which sections you think you already have a good grasp on, and which need review. While you are studying, skim quickly through the familiar sections and take more time on the challenging parts.

Write out your plan so you don't get lost as you go. Having a written plan also helps you feel more in control of the study, so anxiety is less likely to arise from feeling overwhelmed at the amount to cover.

STEP 3: GATHER YOUR TOOLS

Decide what study method works best for you. Do you prefer to highlight in the book as you study and then go back over the highlighted portions? Or do you type out notes of the important information? Or is it helpful to make flashcards that you can carry with you? Assemble the pens, index cards, highlighters, post-it notes, and any other materials you may need so you won't be distracted by getting up to find things while you study.

If you're having a hard time retaining the information or organizing your notes, experiment with different methods. For example, try color-coding by subject with colored pens, highlighters, or post-it notes. If you learn better by hearing, try recording yourself reading your notes so you can listen while in the car, working out, or simply sitting at your desk. Ask a friend to quiz you from your flashcards, or try teaching someone the material to solidify it in your mind.

STEP 4: CREATE YOUR ENVIRONMENT

It's important to avoid distractions while you study. This includes both the obvious distractions like visitors and the subtle distractions like an uncomfortable chair (or a too-comfortable couch that makes you want to fall asleep). Set up the best study environment possible: good lighting and a comfortable work area. If background music helps you focus, you may want to turn it on, but otherwise keep the room quiet. If you are using a computer to take notes, be sure you don't have any other windows open, especially applications like social media, games, or anything else that could distract you. Silence your phone and turn off notifications. Be sure to keep water close by so you stay hydrated while you study (but avoid unhealthy drinks and snacks).

Also, take into account the best time of day to study. Are you freshest first thing in the morning? Try to set aside some time then to work through the material. Is your mind clearer in the afternoon or evening? Schedule your study session then. Another method is to study at the same time of day that you will take the test, so that your brain gets used to working on the material at that time and will be ready to focus at test time.

STEP 5: STUDY!

Once you have done all the study preparation, it's time to settle into the actual studying. Sit down, take a few moments to settle your mind so you can focus, and begin to follow your study plan. Don't give in to distractions or let yourself procrastinate. This is your time to prepare so you'll be ready to fearlessly approach the test. Make the most of the time and stay focused.

Of course, you don't want to burn out. If you study too long you may find that you're not retaining the information very well. Take regular study breaks. For example, taking five minutes out of every hour to walk briskly, breathing deeply and swinging your arms, can help your mind stay fresh.

As you get to the end of each chapter or section, it's a good idea to do a quick review. Remind yourself of what you learned and work on any difficult parts. When you feel that you've mastered the material, move on to the next part. At the end of your study session, briefly skim through your notes again.

But while review is helpful, cramming last minute is NOT. If at all possible, work ahead so that you won't need to fit all your study into the last day. Cramming overloads your brain with more information than it can process and retain, and your tired mind may struggle to recall even previously learned information when it is overwhelmed with last-minute study. Also, the urgent nature of cramming and the stress placed on your brain contribute to anxiety. You'll be more likely to go to the test feeling unprepared and having trouble thinking clearly.

So don't cram, and don't stay up late before the test, even just to review your notes at a leisurely pace. Your brain needs rest more than it needs to go over the information again. In fact, plan to finish your studies by noon or early afternoon the day before the test. Give your brain the rest of the day to relax or focus on other things, and get a good night's sleep. Then you will be fresh for the test and better able to recall what you've studied.

STEP 6: TAKE A PRACTICE TEST

Many courses offer sample tests, either online or in the study materials. This is an excellent resource to check whether you have mastered the material, as well as to prepare for the test format and environment.

Check the test format ahead of time: the number of questions, the type (multiple choice, free response, etc.), and the time limit. Then create a plan for working through them. For example, if you have 30 minutes to take a 60-question test, your limit is 30 seconds per question. Spend less time on the questions you know well so that you can take more time on the difficult ones.

If you have time to take several practice tests, take the first one open book, with no time limit. Work through the questions at your own pace and make sure you fully understand them. Gradually work up to taking a test under test conditions: sit at a desk with all study materials put away and set a timer. Pace yourself to make sure you finish the test with time to spare and go back to check your answers if you have time.

After each test, check your answers. On the questions you missed, be sure you understand why you missed them. Did you misread the question (tests can use tricky wording)? Did you forget the information? Or was it something you hadn't learned? Go back and study any shaky areas that the practice tests reveal.

Taking these tests not only helps with your grade, but also aids in combating test anxiety. If you're already used to the test conditions, you're less likely to worry about it, and working through tests until you're scoring well gives you a confidence boost. Go through the practice tests until you feel comfortable, and then you can go into the test knowing that you're ready for it.

Test Tips

On test day, you should be confident, knowing that you've prepared well and are ready to answer the questions. But aside from preparation, there are several test day strategies you can employ to maximize your performance.

First, as stated before, get a good night's sleep the night before the test (and for several nights before that, if possible). Go into the test with a fresh, alert mind rather than staying up late to study.

Try not to change too much about your normal routine on the day of the test. It's important to eat a nutritious breakfast, but if you normally don't eat breakfast at all, consider eating just a protein bar. If you're a coffee drinker, go ahead and have your normal coffee. Just make sure you time it so that the caffeine doesn't wear off right in the middle of your test. Avoid sugary beverages, and drink enough water to stay hydrated but not so much that you need a restroom break 10 minutes into the test. If your test isn't first thing in the morning, consider going for a walk or doing a light workout before the test to get your blood flowing.

Allow yourself enough time to get ready, and leave for the test with plenty of time to spare so you won't have the anxiety of scrambling to arrive in time. Another reason to be early is to select a good seat. It's helpful to sit away from doors and windows, which can be distracting. Find a good seat, get out your supplies, and settle your mind before the test begins.

When the test begins, start by going over the instructions carefully, even if you already know what to expect. Make sure you avoid any careless mistakes by following the directions.

Then begin working through the questions, pacing yourself as you've practiced. If you're not sure on an answer, don't spend too much time on it, and don't let it shake your confidence. Either skip it and come back later, or eliminate as many wrong answers as possible and guess among the remaining ones. Don't dwell on these questions as you continue—put them out of your mind and focus on what lies ahead.

Be sure to read all of the answer choices, even if you're sure the first one is the right answer. Sometimes you'll find a better one if you keep reading. But don't second-guess yourself if you do immediately know the answer. Your gut instinct is usually right. Don't let test anxiety rob you of the information you know.

If you have time at the end of the test (and if the test format allows), go back and review your answers. Be cautious about changing any, since your first instinct tends to be correct, but make sure you didn't misread any of the questions or accidentally mark the wrong answer choice. Look over any you skipped and make an educated guess.

At the end, leave the test feeling confident. You've done your best, so don't waste time worrying about your performance or wishing you could change anything. Instead, celebrate the successful completion of this test. And finally, use this test to learn how to deal with anxiety even better next time.

> **Review Video: Test Anxiety**
> Visit mometrix.com/academy and enter code: 100340

Important Qualification

Not all anxiety is created equal. If your test anxiety is causing major issues in your life beyond the classroom or testing center, or if you are experiencing troubling physical symptoms related to your anxiety, it may be a sign of a serious physiological or psychological condition. If this sounds like your situation, we strongly encourage you to seek professional help.

Additional Bonus Material

Due to our efforts to try to keep this book to a manageable length, we've created a link that will give you access to all of your additional bonus material:

mometrix.com/bonus948/danboa